Bullying
Among Older Adults

How to Recognize and
Address an Unseen Epidemic

by

Robin P. Bonifas, Ph.D., M.S.W.

with invited contributors

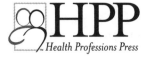

Baltimore • London • Sydney

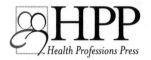

Health Professions Press, Inc.
Post Office Box 10624
Baltimore, Maryland 21285-0624

www.healthpropress.com

Manufactured in the United States of America by Versa Press, East Peoria, Illinois.

All of the cases and examples in this book are composites of the author's actual experiences. In all instances, names have been changed; in some instances, identifying details have been altered to further protect confidentiality.

Library of Congress Cataloging-in-Publication Data

Names: Bonifas, Robin P., author.
Title: Bullying among older adults : how to recognize and address an unseen epidemic / by Robin P. Bonifas, with invited contributors.
Description: Baltimore : Health Professions Press, Inc., [2016] | Includes bibliographical references and index.
Identifiers: LCCN 2016021001 (print) | LCCN 2016021945 (ebook) | ISBN 9781938870095 (pbk.) | ISBN 9781938870484 (epub)
Subjects: | MESH: Bullying—prevention & control | Aged—psychology | Behavior Control—methods | Caregivers
Classification: LCC BF637.B85 (print) | LCC BF637.B85 (ebook) | NLM BF 637.B85 | DDC 302.34/30846—dc23
LC record available at https://lccn.loc.gov/2016021001

British Library Cataloguing-in-Publication data are available from the British Library.

Bullying Among Older Adults

Contents

Downloadable Resources

DOWNLOAD

The following resources are available for download at www.healthpropress.com/bonifas-downloads (use password [case sensitive]: hJZ&sS7n).

About the Author

Robin P. Bonifas, Ph.D., M.S.W., is Associate Professor and Associate Director for Curriculum & Instruction at the Arizona State University School of Social Work. Dr. Bonifas earned her doctorate from the University of Washington in Seattle and has more than 15 years of experience working with older adults and their families in both long-term care and inpatient psychiatric settings. Her research focuses on enhancing psychosocial care for persons with chronic illness and disability, especially those with comorbid mental health conditions and those requiring long-term care. She also evaluates curricular interventions designed to prepare students for effective practice with older adults. Her current projects examine elder social justice issues, such as resident-to-resident aggressive behaviors in nursing homes, bullying among older adults, and other challenges to social relationships in senior care environments. In addition, she is examining the impact of interprofessional education on students' competencies for collaborative healthcare practice.

After completing her master's degree in social work, Dr. Bonifas served as the director of social services in three different skilled nursing facilities over the course of 13 years. She appreciated interacting with individuals in nursing homes so much that she began working on her doctoral degree in 2001 in order eventually to prepare other social workers for practice in this area and to conduct research to advance the field of gerontological social work. The John A. Hartford Foundation funded her doctoral research, which focused on examining factors associated with quality psychosocial care in skilled nursing facilities. Since completing her Ph.D. in 2007, Dr. Bonifas has been working within an academic setting and has continued with research based in skilled nursing as well as the study of social relationship challenges in assisted living.

To date, Dr. Bonifas has given more than 25 presentations across the United States on bullying among older adults, helping senior care providers understand what it is and why it may occur, how it impacts older adults, and what strategies can be used to minimize its occurrence. Her research on resident-to-resident aggression in nursing homes has been published in *Health and Social Work* and the *Journal of the American Medical Directors' Association*.

Dr. Bonifas was named the John A. Hartford Faculty Scholar in Geriatric Social Work in 2011. She serves as the Vice President of the Association of Gerontology Education in Social Work and as a consulting editor for *Health and Social Work* and the *Journal of Gerontological Social Work*. She is also the treasurer for the Arizona chapter of the National Association of Social Workers.

About the Contributors

Eleanor Feldman Barbera, Ph.D., is an accomplished speaker and consultant with nearly 20 years of experience as a psychologist in long-term care. Dr. Barbera writes extensively about mental health issues in long-term care. She is the award-winning author of *The Savvy Resident's Guide* and *McKnight's Long-Term Care News* column "The World According to Dr. El." She combines her training, clinical expertise, and knowledge of the business of long-term care with humor and pragmatism to offer effective solutions to common problems affecting cost and quality of care. Visit Dr. El at MyBetterNursingHome.com for resources to create long-term care settings where everyone thrives.

Katherine Parker Cardinal, M.A., has a master's in Management of Aging Services from the University of Massachusetts, Boston. Her final project, which won the 2015 Management of Aging Services Capstone Award, highlights how evidence-based school bullying prevention and intervention has application in aging services.

As a gerontologist, Cardinal's work demonstrates how community leaders must view social wellness and emotional climate as a responsibility within their power of influence. Synthesizing information across various disciplines, she invites social scientists to study links between social bullying and physical aggression and to explore the complex nature of bullying that co-occurs with emotional or spiritual abuse, mental illness, and substance abuse and within the contexts of racism, homophobia, sexism, and bigotry. She continues to explore the interconnections between childhood trauma, bullying, and unconscious teaching or parenting styles that have been embedded in culture and influenced by centuries-old institutions.

Cardinal credits the pioneering work of Dr. Robin Bonifas, the groundbreaking research of Dan Olweus and Rosalind Wiseman on school bullying, the family-of-origin substance abuse work of John Bradshaw, and her nearly two decades at Project Return in Connecticut working with adolescents challenged by trauma histories for contributing to her understanding of bullying as a lifespan abuse issue that must be properly understood by top management in every senior program and care setting.

Stephanie Langer, J.D., currently practices law through her own practice, Langer Law, P.A., in Coral Gables, Florida. She received her law degree in 1998 from The Catholic University of America, Columbus School of Law, in Washington, D.C., and began her legal career in 1998 in the Miami Dade County State Attorney's Office as an Assistant State Attorney. As a prosecutor, she handled several elder abuse cases. Langer spent 9 years working in private practice litigating cases involving disability discrimination, civil rights violations, fair housing issues, employment discrimination, and education in administrative, state, and federal courts. She also litigated several discrimination cases that involved older adults. Prior to establishing her private practice, Langer had the prestigious honor of working for 2 years at the Southern Poverty Law Center as a staff attorney focused primarily on state-wide education issues. She currently represents older adults in estate planning, guardianship, and probate litigation.

Alyse November, M.S.W., L.C.S.W., earned her master's degree from Adelphi University in New York. She has been in practice since 1989 and has extensive experience working with people of all ages in a variety of settings, including hospitals, schools, hospice, and homecare agencies.

In 2007, November founded Different Like Me, Inc., an agency that employs independent licensed clinical social workers who provide both in-office and in-home psychotherapy services to clients in Palm Beach and Broward counties in Florida with a specialization in the elderly population. She has also created a web-based learning platform called Different Like Me Culture, which offers hands-on interactive learning tools that focus on issues related to bullying for children, adults, and seniors. The senior bullying program is called Senior Culture and focuses on prevention and intervention practices for both older adults and care staff.

In 2012, along with her partner and husband Dr. Steven Essig, November founded Brain Lane Memory Center, LLC, a company that provides both in-home and in-office evaluations, cognitive rehabilitation, behavioral interventions, psychotherapy, resource planning, and education to clients and their families who have been affected by memory disorders. The company's office is located in Delray Beach, Florida.

Jamie Valderrama, M.A., is a lecturer at Arizona State University in the School of Social Work working within the Integrative Health Initiative. She holds a bachelor's in Biology Education and a master's in

Interdisciplinary Studies with an emphasis on integrative health modalities. She trains K–12 teachers and Arizona State University faculty in the effective transfer of knowledge within their courses. She was a public high school teacher for more than 12 years prior to her position with Arizona State University and was named teacher of the year for her high school and district in 2009 and went on to be named an Ambassador of Excellence for the state of Arizona in 2010. In addition to teaching and training, Valderrama conducts keynotes and workshops nationally and internationally on effective teaching practices and the benefits of mindfulness both in and out of the classroom.

Preface

Serving as a nursing assistant in a skilled nursing facility as a teenager, I learned that although the work was tremendously difficult, it was also tremendously rewarding. Furthermore, I loved working with older adults! This was my introduction to gerontology and ultimately shaped the rest of my professional career.

In 2010, while examining resident-to-resident aggression in skilled nursing facilities, I interviewed staff members about the range of negative interactions that occurred among residents. I learned about a phenomenon that contributed to significant emotional distress for facility residents, yet did not meet the definition of actual resident-to-resident aggression. Residents were ridiculing one another, spreading rumors about other residents, and attempting to exclude some residents from group activities. These behaviors reminded me of bullying behaviors common among children and youth in school environments and represented social interaction patterns that had not surfaced in my earlier experiences in skilled nursing facilities.

In discussing these behaviors with a newspaper reporter, the phenomenon was coined "senior bullying." Further media outreach revealed that many seniors across the United States were experiencing problematic peer interactions consistent with bullying in a variety of settings, including senior centers, retirement housing, congregate meal sites, and assisted living facilities. Surprisingly, these incidents appeared to be causing even more emotional distress for older people than the verbal and physical aggression I was studying. Although bullying behaviors were known to exist in a variety of senior living and senior care organizations, minimal research had been conducted on the phenomenon; thus, it was not well understood. I decided I could best advance psychosocial care for older people by extending my research on resident-to-resident aggression to include senior bullying and launched a study of two assisted living facilities to examine these behaviors systematically.

The research occurred in three phases. First, interviews were conducted with 30 individuals residing in assisted living who self-identified as experiencing difficult social interactions with their co-resident peers. Participants were asked about the type of peer behaviors they found most problematic, how the behaviors affected them, the extent of distress they experienced, and how they coped with the behaviors. Second, as part of a follow-up interview, participants completed standardized assessments to help determine the connections between the level of distress associated with negative peer interactions or bullying and cognitive impairment, mood, self-esteem, and the extent of lifetime trauma. Facility staff helped distinguish participants who were bullied from those who were bullied and who also bullied others, so that differences between these two types of targets could be examined. The final stage involved sharing the results with residents and helping them to develop a resident-driven intervention to minimize bullying. The results of this research are featured extensively in this book and provide a foundation of empirical evidence for the range of bullying behaviors that tend to occur among older adults and the impact of such experiences on emotional well-being.

Once the media reported the findings of this research, numerous senior care providers contacted me to share the incredible difficulties they have experienced trying to manage bullying and other antagonistic behaviors among older adults in their organizations. Older adults themselves called me, sent e-mails, and mailed letters describing their negative experiences with other older adults. Over and over, providers and seniors alike expressed an intense need for guidance in how to effectively minimize such behaviors.

This book was written to address the need to understand bullying behaviors among older adults and pulls together promising interventions suggested by my research and developed by my colleagues who contributed to this book and who, like me, share a deep concern for the psychosocial well-being of older adults.

Note that the term *target* is used throughout this book rather than *victim* to reinforce the idea that people need not be passive recipients of such hurtful behavior. Care providers can be trained to recognize and minimize bullying behaviors, and those who are bullied can be taught effective skills to address and even prevent such behaviors.

It is my hope that this book will extend the reach of this vital information to more individuals who are positioned to improve social relationship experiences for more older adults.

PART I

An Overview of Bullying Behaviors Among Older Adults

CHAPTER 1

An Introduction to Bullying Behaviors Among Older Adults

~~~~~~

"He calls me 'fatso.' He says, 'Hey fatso.'
Then as he goes down the hall . . . he makes oinking
noises [like a pig] as he goes to the elevator."

This comment, and others like it, was made by a 72-year-old resident of an assisted living facility (Bonifas, 2011). His target, a 78-year-old woman, had heard similar comments from this individual for more than a year, beginning shortly after she moved into the facility. These repetitive negative remarks about her body size lowered her self-esteem and contributed to self-isolation; she reported reluctance to leave her room for fear of being ridiculed by the individual, whom she referred to as a "bully." The incidents this woman experienced represent relational aggression, a form of bullying common among older adults in communal living settings and congregate service organizations.

People who rarely interact with older adults often erroneously perceive that the population is composed primarily of sweet little grandmas and grandpas who get along well with one another. Accordingly, many people are surprised to learn that bullying behaviors actually occur among older adults. Indeed, they do. Although bullying is commonly associated with youth in school settings, research and media reports indicate that such behaviors are common as well among older adults. For example, up to 20% of older adults in assisted living facilities (Bonifas & Kramer, 2011; Trompetter,

3

Scholte, & Westerhof, 2011) and 50% in independent retirement settings (Benson, 2012) report having experienced some form of peer bullying. A pilot study to begin understanding bullying behaviors among older adults revealed that 28 of 30 assisted living residents interviewed had experienced bullying or other negative peer social interactions since moving into their facility, and all had witnessed other residents endure bullying behaviors (Bonifas, 2011).

Contrary to the childhood adage, "Sticks and stones may break my bones, but names will never hurt me," exposure to bullying behaviors contributes to emotional distress for both the targets and the witnesses, as well as detracts from a positive sense of community in senior living and senior care organizations. (Note that the term *target* is used throughout this book rather than *victim* to reinforce the idea that people who are bullied can prevent bullying incidents by learning effective skills and need not be passive victims of hurtful behavior.) For example, older adults who reported being bullied by peers within the preceding year scored higher on measures of depression and lower on measures of self-esteem compared to their counterparts who did not report bullying experiences (Bonifas, 2011). Similarly, they indicated that preexisting mental health conditions were often exacerbated by exposure to bullying. Witnesses to bullying behaviors experienced distress and feelings of helplessness when they saw their peers being picked on. Not knowing how to intervene, they avoided getting involved and then felt shame that they did not make an effort to stop the negative interactions. Furthermore, the overall negative climate created by bullying contributes to dissatisfaction with one's living situation and an increased focus on moving out (personal communication, Marsha Frankel, March 30, 2011).

Staff members also experience distress in settings where bullying and other negative interactions occur among older adults. These staff, who strive to create a pleasant living environment, are being thwarted by bullying behaviors among the individuals in their care. For example, one continuing care retirement community dedicated to desegregating residents by level of care experienced ongoing tensions between comingled independent living residents and assisted living residents. The higher-functioning independent residents were very vocal about not wanting to associate with the lower-functioning assisted living residents (personal communication, Alyse November, September 5, 2015).

Addressing bullying behaviors among older adults is critically important to enhancing quality of life and promoting emotional well-being for both residents and staff in senior living and care settings. This chapter begins to explore the issue by first defining the types of bullying that occur among older adults.

Bullying Defined

Bullying is intentional repetitive aggressive behavior that involves an imbalance of power or strength (Hazelden Foundation, 2011). Associated peer bullying extends beyond this to include the experience of "persistent negative interpersonal behavior" (Rayner & Keashly, 2005, p. 271) that is directed at a specific individual or a group of individuals (Rayner & Keashly, 2005). As noted earlier, among older adults, such negative behaviors often take the form of relational bullying, which represents nonphysical aggression intended to hinder the formation of peer relationships and social connections (Hawker & Boulton, 2000), such as gossiping, spreading rumors, and public ridiculing.

Surprisingly, bullying among older adults looks similar in many ways to bullying among younger age groups. For example, both include verbal, physical, and antisocial or relational behaviors that occur in the context of social relationships in communal settings. Furthermore, the individual targets of bullies at any age suffer considerable emotional anguish.

Types of Bullying

The following sections review the characteristics of three types of bullying behaviors among older adults: verbal, antisocial or relational, and physical.

Verbal Bullying

Verbal bullying refers to the use of words to intimidate or otherwise usurp another's power. Behaviors include name-calling, malicious teasing, hurling insults, taunting, threatening, or making sarcastic remarks or pointed jokes. An example of verbal bullying is the name-calling experienced by the 78-year-old woman introduced in the chapter's opening. As another example, George, a resident of an assisted living facility, described threatening remarks he regularly endured from another resident: "There's one that tries to be the number one tough guy. [He comes up] to me [and says] 'One of these days, I'm gonna smack you with a hammer.'" Although it was unknown whether the individual making this threat actually had a hammer and intended to follow through with his violent action, having this statement directed at him again and again caused George significant ongoing anxiety. This worry was magnified by their random nature; George could not predict when they would occur or identify what might have triggered the threats.

Antisocial or Relational Bullying

Antisocial or relational bullying involves behaviors, either verbal or nonverbal, that are intended to hinder another's social relationships or limit social connections. Examples include shunning, excluding or ignoring, gossiping, mimicking someone's walk or disability, making offensive gestures or facial expressions, purposely turning one's head or body away when the target speaks, using threatening body language, or purposefully encroaching on personal space. Paula, a resident of a senior housing community, explains: "I would describe bullying like harassment . . . [it's not] just pushing and shoving and fighting all the time . . . [it] includes harassment, like if you want to go through the door and someone [purposefully] stands in your way" (personal communication, April 8, 2014). Another resident, John, was shunned by other residents. After relocating to senior housing in another state following the loss of his home during Hurricane Katrina, several residents of John's new apartment complex began spreading rumors that he was a longtime homeless man and was the first in a deluge of formerly homeless people who were going to be "dumped" into their building. As a result, other residents began to avoid John (Bonifas & Frankel, 2012).

Physical Bullying

Physical bullying involves actual bodily contact with the target or the target's belongings, including pets or personal possessions. Example behaviors include pushing, hitting, kicking, destroying property, or stealing. Hitting might be with a hand, closed fist, or mobility aid, such as a cane. In 2012, *ABC News* reported on 71-year-old Bernadine Jones' experiences of being bullied by her 87-year-old neighbor, Maria Zuravinski. A resident of a senior housing community, Ms. Jones said she was working in the community's garden one day when "Zuravinski approached her . . . and accused her of disturbing some of her personal plants . . . the confrontation escalated when Zuravinski began yelling at her and calling her names and then hit her with her cane and spat on her" (Reese, 2012, p. 2). Ms. Jones continued to be subjected to similar behaviors from her neighbor. At one point, Ms. Zuravinski even attempted to strike Ms. Jones' dog with her cane. Ms. Jones reported feeling so distressed by her neighbor's behavior that she was "afraid to go out [her] door." She explained, "I have to look out before I leave" (Reese, 2012, p. 2).

The Emotional Impact of Bullying Behaviors Among Older Adults

Individuals who are the targets of bullying are significantly affected by their peers' negative behaviors. Among older adults, verbal and antisocial bullying are more common than physical violence, but all types of bullying have negative effects on those who experience them as well as those who witness them. For example, one assisted living resident described how he would be kept up at night by other residents yelling at one another, not only because of the noise disruption, but also because of his fears of potential escalating violence. He stated, "It is the uncertainty of what [they] are going to do that I find most unsettling" (Bonifas, 2011).

Common responses to bullying behaviors among older adults include the following (items 1 through 7 from Bonifas [2011], and items 8 through 14 from Bonifas & Frankel [2012]):

1. anger/annoyance

2. intense frustration

3. fearfulness

4. anxiety/tension/worry

5. retaliation followed by shame

6. self-isolation

7. exacerbation of mental health conditions

8. reduced self-esteem

9. overall feelings of rejection

10. depressive symptoms, including changes in eating and sleeping

11. increased physical complaints

12. functional changes, such as decreased ability to manage activities of daily living

13. increased talk of moving out

14. suicidal ideation

Staff and family care partners should watch for these emotional effects as indications that someone is potentially being bullied.

Bullying behaviors also negatively affect senior living communities as a whole. For example, bullying among residents can contribute to pervasive feelings of fear, disrespect, and insecurity; perpetuate more bullying behaviors; and lead to lowered resident satisfaction and reduced involvement in planned group activities (personal communication, Marsha Frankel, March 14, 2014). Although research has yet to be conducted on the organizational implications of bullying among older adults, anecdotal evidence provided by Frankel suggests that working in a senior living or senior care environment where bullying and other negative social behaviors occur regularly contributes to low employee morale and poor job satisfaction. These outcomes can lead to decreased feelings of loyalty and commitment to the organization and, ultimately, costly staff turnover. Furthermore, Frankel notes that the possibility of staff bullying residents in retaliation for peer bullying or even of abusing residents in their care may increase due to feelings of frustration and anger. The potential for such negative outcomes is magnified when staff members feel unable to take steps to reduce the bullying behaviors, either because they do not know how or because efforts are repeatedly ineffective. Thus, equipping staff with skills to effectively address bullying is critical to minimize negative outcomes. Chapter 7 provides a detailed intervention to teach long-term care staff how to thwart bullying incidents.

It is important to remember that family members and other visitors to senior organizations may witness bullying behaviors as well. Such occurrences can contribute to family concerns regarding the quality of the facility as well as their loved one's physical safety and emotional well-being. There is currently no evidence that links the existence of bullying behaviors to poor care or unmet resident needs; indeed, some experts have suggested that bullying is likely to occur to some extent in all senior living settings (American Senior Housing Association, 2014). However, evidence does suggest that such problematic interactions are less common in organizations that promote an atmosphere of caring and respect among both residents and staff as well as where residents are engaged and active in numerous events and projects. Strategies to create such environments are presented in Chapters 7, 8, and 9.

Distinguishing Bullying from Challenging Behavior in General

Although many behaviors exhibited by older adults can be challenging, the situation in which the behavior occurs and the type of behavior often determine whether it is actually bullying versus a challenging behavior whereby a resident is simply being rude or unpleasant. Key factors that define an incident as bullying include behaviors that (1) are directed at a specific person or group of people, (2) involve an imbalance of power or a desire to gain power, or (3) occur repeatedly in most cases. The phrase "in most cases" is used here because there is evidence of one-time episodes of bullying contributing to significant emotional distress for some individuals, a phenomenon that is discussed further at the end of this chapter.

As an example of a challenging behavior that does not meet the definition of bullying, consider an individual who yells and strikes out at most everyone in his or her environment. This is not necessarily bullying because the behavior does not target a specific individual or group of individuals. Similarly, a behavior may be inappropriate and violate community rules, but is not truly bullying because the dynamics of power and control are absent. For example, in a public area of an assisted living facility a resident showing visible symptoms of mental illness, such as engaging in loud and animated conversations with unseen stimuli, may frighten and upset other residents. His behavior, however, is not motivated by a need for power over others, is not interpersonal, and is not directed at anyone specifically. As a further example, two individuals with strong personalities who frequently butt heads over differences of opinion are not engaging in bullying even if verbally abusive language and negative gestures are used because they are equally matched; one is not able to use his or her power to control or intimidate the other. However, if one of these individuals is more timid and is being pressured to join the other's side or face exclusion, then bullying is occurring. The term *power* refers to inner personal strength in influencing others to align with one's point of view. In the context of bullying, personal power is used negatively to harm others physically, emotionally, or socially.

Activity 1.1 allows readers to test their knowledge of the differences between bullying and challenging behaviors. Try to determine whether each scenario is bullying or not and why, then review the answers to see if you were correct.

It is important to keep in mind that some people exhibit verbal or physical aggression when they are frustrated or upset as a way of communicating their feelings, especially those in the advanced stages of dementia. In these cases, the behaviors do not stem from a need to domineer and control others, but instead are due to brain deterioration and associated difficulty in accurately perceiving and effectively responding to environmental stimuli. Such behaviors require alternative modes of intervention that address impulse control challenges, communication difficulties, frustration regarding impaired task performance, and misperceptions of potential environmental threats. (Visit the Alzheimer's Association website for excellent resources on behavioral management in dementia [www.alz.org].) In these instances, however, it is important to remember that exposure to such unpleasant or disruptive behaviors can feel like bullying to the person experiencing the behaviors. Activity 1.2 identifies common peer behaviors viewed as most distressing to residents in assisted living (Bonifas & Kramer, 2011). Readers can use the activity to test their knowledge of which behaviors are bullying and which are simply challenging behaviors.

The intentional nature of bullying may not be as relevant for older adults as it is for other age groups. In some older adults,

ACTIVITY 1.1

Is It Bullying?

Scenario 1: An older woman yells loudly several times in a congregate meal setting filled with other older adults that she does not like the chair she is sitting in. Is she being a bully?

Scenario 2: A resident in an assisted living facility repeatedly tells another resident who is foreign-born that he will see to it that she is evicted because she cannot speak English properly. Is he being a bully?

Answers: Scenario 1 is not bullying. The behavior is not directed at a specific individual or group of individuals and does not appear to stem from a need to dominate others. If, instead, the older woman encroached on another resident's personal space and loudly yelled at him "Get out of my chair or I will throw this coffee on you!" the situation would be bullying.

Scenario 2 is bullying. The behavior is targeted at a specific individual and is intended to intimidate her. It would even be bullying if he had said, "You people over there at the card table who can't speak English properly need to leave." Alternatively, if the individual had yelled out in the community room "People who can't speak proper English should leave!" it would not be considered bullying because the behavior is not directed toward a specific individual or group of individuals.

particularly for those with cognitive loss, merely the perception that a peer means to bully or interact negatively can contribute to a feeling of victimization. This phenomenon is described in greater detail in Chapter 6. Some scholars have recognized that lay individuals may define bullying somewhat differently than researchers and professionals (Liefooghe & Mackenzie Davey, 2003; Saunders, Huynh, & Goodman-Delahunty, 2007) Indeed, Altman (2010) indicates that Novak's (1998) theory of learning draws attention to the influence of perception, whereby individuals assign meaning to behavior based on past experiences and preexisting knowledge. To illustrate this complex explanation, consider the experience of an assisted living resident who is exposed to another resident's psychiatric symptoms stemming from combat-related post-traumatic stress disorder. Imagine such an individual, who has never been exposed to this type of behavior in the past, observing and hearing his peer engage in loud

ACTIVITY 1.2

Is It Bullying?

Check your knowledge of which of these are bullying behaviors or challenging behaviors. See the answers in the note below.

- Exposure to loud arguments in communal areas
- Being the focus of naming-calling and disparaging remarks
- Being the focus of gossiping and rumor-spreading
- Being bossed around or told what to do
- Negotiating value differences, especially related to diversity of beliefs stemming from differences in culture, spirituality, or socioeconomic status
- Competing for scarce resources, especially seating, television programming in communal areas, and staff attention
- Being harassed to loan money, cigarettes, or other commodities
- Not being able to avoid listening to others complain
- Experiencing physical aggression
- Witnessing psychiatric symptoms, especially those that are frightening or disruptive

---

Bullying behaviors include: being the focus of name-calling and disparaging remarks; being the focus of gossiping and rumor-spreading; being bossed around or told what to do; being harassed to loan money, cigarettes, or other commodities; and experiencing physical aggression.

animated conversations with unseen stimuli that include phrases like "take out the enemy," "concentrated gunfire," and "massive aerial attack." With no context to understand these behaviors, the individual may perceive them as highly frightening and disruptive as well as personally directed at him. As a result, he may mistakenly label his peer a bully (Bonifas & Kramer, 2011). This type of misunderstanding can also happen in skilled nursing facilities when individuals feel as if their personal space is being invaded by peers with dementia who wander: although the invasive behavior stems from cognitive impairments rather than malicious intent, they still report feeling purposefully targeted by those individuals.

A single episode of exposure to negative interpersonal behavior can also be perceived as bullying among older adults (Olweus, 1993). In Chapter 8, Alyse November shares the story of a couple living in independent senior housing who were shunned the first time they sought seating in the dining room and never returned to have meals there. As another example, the following letter to the editor illustrates the distress associated with a one-time incident:

Unwelcoming Reception at Middletown Bingo

Dear Editor,

I am appalled at the seniors at the Middletown Senior Center in Silverdale that I met when I tried to attend bingo. I lived in Silverdale all through the late 70s and the 80s and had nice neighbors and friends. After returning to this area following 20 years in California, I decided to go to bingo at the Middletown Senior Center to see if I would know anyone. I was treated very rudely, to say the least. These women lied to me at every single table where I tried to sit down at one of the several empty seats without coats, cards, coffee, or purses. I was not even allowed to pull up a chair on the end, as I was told that there would be no room for my cards once the chairs were filled. They were the most unfriendly, unwelcoming, mean, and rude group of women I have ever met. There was no one sitting in those seats and they lied that they were taken (I was 40 minutes early to be sure to get a good seat). Shame on you, mean people, and what you did to a kind lady who was thinking of offering to volunteer at the center. You are a disgrace to your community.

Sincerely,
Mrs. Underwood

Distinguishing Between Bullying and Elder Abuse

In contrast to bullying, *elder abuse* is defined as any knowing, intended, or careless act that causes harm or serious risk of harm to an older person, whether physical, mental, emotional, or financial (National Center on Elder Abuse [NCEA], 2011). Elder abuse also includes the knowing deprivation by a caregiver of goods or services necessary to meet the elder's essential needs or to avoid physical or psychological harm (NCEA, 2006). As with bullying, there are several types of elder abuse: physical, sexual, emotional, psychological, and verbal abuse, as well as neglect and exploitation. Although elder abuse and bullying are distinct phenomena with separate definitions, the two are not mutually exclusive; sometimes bullying and abuse can intersect. Both can include hitting, kicking, pinching, yelling, threats, humiliation, or ridicule.

In order to properly distinguish between bullying and elder abuse, one must consider who is engaging in the negative behavior or aggressive act and who is the target of the behavior. With elder abuse, the target is a vulnerable adult, someone who is dependent on another for personal care or instrumental assistance, such as bathing or financial management. With bullying, both the bully and the target of bullying are vulnerable adults, and the target is not dependent on the bully for any type of care or assistance. The examples in Table 1.1 illustrate the differences among elder abuse, bullying, nonbullying behaviors, and challenging behaviors in older adults.

It is crucial to recognize that bullying can escalate to physical violence. For example, in September 2009, Elizabeth Barrow, a 100-year-old nursing home resident, was killed by her 98-year-old roommate, Laura Lindquist, after ongoing misperceptions of

Table 1.1. Comparison and contrast of elder abuse, bullying, nonbullying behaviors, and challenging behaviors

Elder abuse	Mickey Rooney, 90-year-old film and television star, reported feeling powerless when his stepson took and misused his money and withheld food and medicine from him (Anderson, 2011).
Bullying	Edward, an assisted living resident, voiced feeling reluctant to leave his room to attend activities of interest because a fellow resident, Craig, continually pressured him for money and threatened to knock him down if he refused to loan him any (Bonifas, 2011).
Nonbullying behaviors	Esther, an assisted living resident, often asked her tablemates for spare change so she could buy items from the vending machines, but she didn't pressure them. Although her tablemates felt slightly irritated by her requests, they didn't feel threatened or unable to say no (Bonifas, 2011).
Challenging behaviors	Betty, an attendee at a congregate meal site for older adults, loudly sang The Lord's Prayer throughout meals, disrupting others' enjoyment of their lunch, but not threatening them in any way. (Bonifas, 2011).

unequal room space and associated feelings of anger (Kessler, 2009). The attorney for Mrs. Barrow reported that during the weeks before her murder, she complained that Mrs. Lindquist "[made] her life a 'living hell'" (p. 1).

Summary

Bullying behaviors among older adults are a significant problem in senior living and care organizations. In her work with senior housing communities in Florida, Alyse November, a licensed clinical social worker and the author of Chapters 8 and 10, has called bullying an "unseen epidemic." Bullying experiences negatively affect older adults (the targets of bullying as well as those who bully), the staff members assisting them, and the milieu of an organization as a whole. Chapter 2 goes on to address the extent of what is known about bullying among older adults as well as bullying among other age groups and how knowledge of bullying across the life span can inform our understanding of being bullied in older adulthood.

Understanding Bullying Among Older Adults

~~~~~~

What Do We Know?

Robin P. Bonifas
Jamie Valderrama

Current Research on Bullying Among Older Adults

Although few studies have examined bullying and other challenging behaviors among older adults, research to date has provided some insights into the phenomenon. For example, we have some knowledge of the types of settings where bullying occurs, situations that contribute to bullying behaviors, general characteristics of older individuals who bully or who are the targets of bullies, and the outcomes of being bullied in older adulthood.

Senior Settings Where Bullying Tends to Occur

Relational aggression and associated indirect forms of bullying are the most common types of bullying among older adults (Benson, 2012; Rex-Lear, 2011; Trompetter, Scholte, & Westerhof, 2011). Research indicates that such behaviors are likely to occur in small social groups composed of members who interact regularly (Bjorkqvist, Ekman, & Lagerspetz, 1982) and who experience difficulty leaving the group if relational aggression occurs

(Smith & Brain, 2000). Senior centers, congregate meal settings, and all forms of senior housing fit the definition of small social groups that have regular social interaction and are difficult to leave. Impediments to leaving include an alternative senior center that may not be convenient to available forms of transportation and the availability of meal services (Pardasani, 2010) that participants may take advantage of daily and that may not be accessible elsewhere.

Situations that Contribute to Senior Bullying

Among older adults, relational aggression tends to be planned and used to counteract negative emotions that arise during interpersonal conflict (Walker & Richardson, 1998). For example, Sarah, a resident of an assisted living facility, felt threatened by Marie because a gentleman she was romantically interested in commented on Marie's attractiveness. Consequently, Sarah would often loudly ridicule Marie's appearance in communal areas in an attempt to mitigate her own feelings of jealousy (Bonifas, 2011).

The wide variety of older adults in a setting can also contribute to challenging social interactions in senior housing and senior centers. Negative interactions may stem from feelings of discomfort with the diversity of values, perspectives, and lifestyles that exist among individuals living or participating in these settings. One assisted living resident, for example, commented that "For me, the hardest part [of being here] has been living with people I have never associated with in my life" (Bonifas, 2011). Another resident stated that "I'm being forced to associate with people that I have nothing in common with and I don't even like . . . I was not prepared for this" (Bonifas, 2011). Both of these comments illustrate the challenges older adults may experience trying to adjust to the diversity of being and thinking that is often present in communal environments. Such difficulties are especially salient when individuals are reluctantly living with unfamiliar people in relatively close quarters where avoiding one another may be challenging unless they also avoid valued community resources, such as group activities or dining services.

Generational differences can also be a factor in difficulties with social relationships, especially in settings that attract both younger people with disabilities and older adults. Members of the American Association of Service Coordinators, who oversee resident affairs in many senior housing organizations, reported during group discussions held at a professional conference that these two groups often do not see eye to eye and tend to antagonize one another (personal communication, August 20, 2013). For example, younger individuals might loudly play music of their era to purposely annoy older co-residents who find it distasteful. Similarly, older residents might negatively comment on the poor values of "kids these days" within earshot of younger co-residents to purposely trigger angry outbursts. In describing this generational divide, one assisted living resident stated that "They go two generations back from me and I have no idea what they're talking about" (Bonifas, 2011). This comment illustrates the level of disconnection felt between different age groups in communal settings.

Pervasive feelings of loss common among older people in senior housing and senior centers can also contribute to negative social interactions. Examples include physical health declines, financial insecurity, reduced productivity, and greater dependence on others for functional assistance (Shinoda–Tagawa et al., 2004). All of these changes can minimize one's sense of control, lead to self-devaluation, and generate negative emotions that detract from healthy social relationships (Nay, 1995). For example, Irene, a resident of an independent senior housing complex, reported feeling devastated by the loss of her prized caregiver role when her husband died and her grandchildren later moved out of state. In an effort to continue her caregiving role in some capacity, she began spontaneously advising the frailer tenants in her building using a bossy communication style, to the point that her co-residents began to see her as a bully.

Individual Characteristics Associated with Bullying Among Older Adults

Engaging in bullying and relationally aggressive behaviors requires a certain level of cognitive and social acuity (Walker & Richardson, 1998). As such, senior living environments with higher functioning residents tend to have more problems with bullying because such individuals possess the necessary memory and organizational skills to engage in planned behaviors. This is evident in Benson's (2012) research on relational aggression in independent senior living communities in which tenants required no hands-on assistance: 50% of residents had experienced at least some peer bullying in the preceding year. This is in large contrast to Bonifas and Kramer's (2011) study of assisted living residents who were somewhat lower functioning and had more cognitive impairments than those in Benson's sample: only 20% of residents experienced peer bullying. Similarly, Rex-Lear (2011) reported that bullying episodes are more frequent among older adults in community settings relative to institutional settings, and Wood (2007) found that most individuals with no cognitive impairments who were living in nursing homes experienced bullying only "now and then" (p. 56). Indeed, among assisted living residents, better performance on the Montreal Cognitive Assessment (MoCA; Nasreddine et al., 2005), a cognitive-testing instrument, was associated with engaging in bullying behaviors while lower performance was associated with not engaging in bullying. On average, individuals who bullied scored 3.44 points higher on the MoCA than their nonbullying peers, placing them in the typical range, whereas those who did not bully often had mild cognitive impairments (Bonifas & Kramer, 2011). This finding provides additional support to the idea that relatively strong cognitive skills are a necessary component of bullying behaviors.

Although this chapter has focused so far on individuals who bully, it is important to note that in communal settings, small groups of like-minded residents sometimes can band together to form cliques that collectively bully or harass others. In assisted living communities, "welcoming committees" are not uncommon. This purposefully oxymoronic term refers to the situation in which a few residents spend most of their day in the facility lobby or other prominent locations observing and making malicious comments toward all who enter and exit the area. Such cliques can also manifest in dining areas and activity groups.

Older Adult Outcomes Associated with Being Bullied

As noted in Chapter 1, exposure to relational aggression contributes to social isolation and intense feelings of anger and fearfulness among residents of assisted living, as well as exacerbates existing physical and mental health conditions (Bonifas & Kramer, 2011). Although no longitudinal studies have been completed to date, cross-sectional research links the experience of relational aggression and bullying in older adulthood to depressive symptoms, low self-esteem, anxiety, social loneliness, and reduced life satisfaction

(Benson, 2012; Bonifas & Hector, 2013; Trompetter et al., 2011). Indeed, Benson (2012) found that depressive symptoms among targets of bullying were nine times higher than for those who did not experience peer bullying. Other outcomes associated with bullying among older adults include poorer physical health, more frequent physical complaints, and higher levels of psychological distress manifested by worry, irritability, and disorganization. These findings were especially pronounced for men and for individuals who had been victimized earlier in life (Rex-Lear, 2011). It is important to remember, however, that these research results are cross-sectional, or measured at one point in time, and, therefore, causation cannot be implied. In other words, it is not evident which comes first, bullying or the negative outcome. For example, rather than relational aggression and bullying causing social loneliness and depressive symptoms, it is equally possible that individuals who are lonely and depressed may be more vulnerable to peer bullying. It is also possible that the influence works both ways, with one phenomenon exacerbating the other in an escalating cycle.

In addition, the harmful effects of bullying are not exclusive to the recipients of such behavior. Individuals who witness bullying also experience negative consequences. Some feel guilty for not intervening, which contributes to a sense of poor self-worth (Marsha Frankel, personal communication, January 26, 2012). Similarly, individuals who do retaliate by reciprocal bullying also report significant feelings of shame that they "stooped to the bully's level" (Bonifas, 2011). For example, Bill, an assisted living resident, described being threatened by Ralph: "He said he would hit me if I didn't change the TV to the stupid ball game. I told him I would break his cane in half if he tried. Later that night, I felt so bad that I had said something so petty and low. Can you imagine threatening to break some old man's cane?"

Current Research on Bullying Among Children and Youth and How It Applies to Older Adults

The following sections detail what is known about bullying in children and young people, which can lend additional insights into peer bullying among older adults.

Factors Associated with Bullying Among Younger People

According to Stopbullying.gov, a website managed by the U.S. Department of Health and Human Services, children and adolescents who exhibit bullying behaviors tend to fall into two categories: (1) a socially popular child who wants to maintain status by dominating others, and (2) a socially isolated child who lacks empathy and struggles with his or her self-esteem who bullies in an effort to increase social status and power. Characteristics that may contribute to bullying behaviors among youth include being more aggressive in general or experiencing any of the following: low frustration tolerance, limited parental involvement, problems or difficulties at home, negative valuation of others, difficulty adhering to rules, viewing violence positively, or belonging to a peer group who bullies (StopBullying.gov).

How might this information apply to older adults who bully? First, if bullying behaviors among youth are triggered by a desire to maintain social status, it is likely that bullying behaviors among older adults may be triggered for the same reason. This aligns with the information presented earlier that bullying behaviors among older adults is often associated with loss, especially loss of valued social roles and the desire to regain some semblance of control. There are numerous situations in which older adults might find their social status threatened: moving into a senior housing setting, joining a new recreational group or social club, or entering into group-based services at a senior center. Such experiences involve introduction to a new peer group, which can be intimidating and lead to a desire to fit in and create a place for oneself in the group. For some individuals, this can create a sense of helplessness and a subsequent need to dominate others in an attempt to foster a feeling of control over one's social position. A similar response can occur when an individual who is socially established in a given setting is confronted with a new addition to the group. This situation can threaten the established individual's position in the setting, leading to bullying or other antagonistic behaviors toward the newcomer in an effort to maintain his or her place in the social hierarchy. The presence of newcomers may stimulate concerns regarding reduced access to scarce desirable resources, resulting in bullying behaviors to maintain control of those assets. For example, in the southwestern states, which are popular wintertime residences for northern "snowbirds," year-long residents may lash out toward seasonal visitors when they feel crowded out from their customary use of space (Maureen McCarthy, personal communication, January 20, 2016).

Among youth, lack of parental involvement is associated with bullying behaviors. Although parental involvement does not apply to older adults, its ramifications can advance understanding of bullying among older people. Youth whose parents are not involved in their lives can feel unappreciated and unloved, resulting in intense feelings of anger or low self-esteem, which can contribute to bullying behaviors in an effort to gain social recognition or a sense of self-efficacy. Correspondingly, older adults who are isolated with minimal connections to family members and friends may have similar feelings and subsequent aggressive reactions toward peers.

In addition to verbal, social or relational, and physical bullying, children and youth also engage in cyberbullying, which involves the use of technology, such as cell phones, computers, and electronic tablets, in addition to social media sites, such as Twitter, Tumbler, Instagram, and Facebook, to send derogatory messages about the target. Disparaging emails or text messages may be directed to an individual child, criticizing his or her appearance or degrading his or her social worth, or communications might be directed to a group in order to humiliate the target by starting negative rumors, often accompanied by embarrassing photos and videos. Cyberbullying is especially challenging because it is difficult for young people to avoid. For example, Stopbullying.gov lists the following characteristics of cyberbullying that hinder the ability to manage it effectively:

- Cyberbullying can happen 24 hours a day, 7 days a week, and reach a [child] even when he or she is alone. It can happen any time of the day or night.
- Cyberbullying messages and images can be posted anonymously and distributed quickly to a very wide audience. It can be difficult and sometimes impossible to trace the source.
- Deleting inappropriate or harassing messages, texts, and pictures is extremely difficult after they have been posted or sent.

Although there is currently no data on the extent of cyberbullying among older adults, the growing use of the Internet and cell phone technology in this population suggests it is likely to be a problem now and in the future. As of 2013, 59% of individuals age 65 and older reported using the Internet and 77% owned a cell phone (Pew Research Center, 2012). The Washington State Office of the Attorney General's website *Internet Safety for Seniors* acknowledges cyberbullying exists among older adults, typically occurs via email in the form of emotional or financial abuse, and is most often perpetrated by family members. It is important for senior care providers to be attuned to this potential problem, especially since use of the Internet and cell phone technology has increased since the Pew Research Center study cited above was conducted.

Factors Associated with Being the Target of Bullying Among Children and Youth

Insights into what is associated with being the target of youth bullying can also facilitate understanding of what creates vulnerability to peer bullying among older people. Among youth targets, some characteristics associated with vulnerability include being perceived as different from others; appearing weak or unable to stand up for oneself; being depressed, anxious, or having low self-esteem; having few friends or being less popular; or having difficulties getting along with others (StopBullying.gov). In addition, gender differences in target characteristics and forms of bullying have been noted among young people. For boys, risk factors linked to being bullied include younger age, having been in a physical fight, being physically inactive, truancy, and psychosocial distress. Predominant forms of bullying are physical and include being hit, kicked, pushed, shoved around, or locked indoors (Pengpid & Peltzer, 2013). For girls, risk factors include having been in a physical fight, lack of parental bonding, and psychosocial distress. Bullying is verbal or social in nature, such as being made fun of with sexual jokes, comments, and gestures (Pengpid & Peltzer, 2013).

These insights suggest that the following types of older people are vulnerable to being bullied by their peers: those who are perceived as being different from the dominant group, unable to defend themselves, or socially isolated, as well as those struggling with feelings of emotional distress (depression, anxiety) or who have low self-esteem. This corresponds to research findings presented in Chapter 3, namely that older adults who report high levels of distress stemming from being bullied by their peers also score higher on measures of depressive symptoms and lower on measures of self-esteem compared to individuals who report minimal levels of distress (Bonifas & Kramer, 2011). This also aligns with Benson's (2012) findings that older adults who use an assistive mobility device are bullied more often than their counterparts who do not. People who bully may view individuals who use a walker, cane, wheelchair, or motorized scooter as being less capable of self-defense. Furthermore, gender differences exist among older targets as well. Indeed, as discussed in Chapter 3, men tend to be more physically aggressive and women tend to be more socially or relationally aggressive (Marsha Frankel, personal communication, March 30, 2013).

Prevalence of Bullying Behaviors Among Children and Youth

The number of young people engaging in and experiencing peer bullying, as well as the frequency of negative behaviors that occur, can provide clues regarding how often older adults are involved in bullying situations and the nature of their involvement. In the United States, research on bullying among adolescents indicates that prevalence rates for the four types of bullying as either an aggressor or a target over a 2-month period were 20.8% for physical behaviors, 53.6% for verbal behaviors, 51.4% for social or relational aggressive behaviors, and 13.6% for cyberbullying (Wang, Iannotti, & Nansel, 2009). During the 2010-2011 academic year, 27.8% of students ages 12–18 experienced bullying (Lessne & Harmalkar, 2013). Consistent with Wang et al.'s findings, the most common forms of peer bullying were being the "subject of rumors" (18.3%), being "made fun of, called names, or insulted" (17.6%), and being "pushed, shoved, tripped, or spit on" (7.9%) (2009, p. 5). Although rates of cyberbullying are relatively low compared to other forms of bullying, specific groups may be at higher risk. For example, research indicates that 55.2% of lesbian, gay, bisexual, or transgender (LGBT) youth ages 13–20 experienced cyberbullying during 2011 (Kosciw, Greytak, Bartkiewicz, Boesen, & Palmer, 2012). These findings suggest that among older adults, verbal and social forms of bullying are likely to be the most common, and physical and cyberbullying likely the least common. Older people perceived as different, and especially those from stigmatized groups, may be more vulnerable to being the targets of bullying. Findings presented in Chapter 1 align with this hypothesis: assisted living residents tended to report verbal and social forms of bullying and antagonistic behaviors (gossiping, rumor spreading, and name calling) as the most challenging types of social interaction patterns compared to physically aggressive actions (Bonifas & Kramer, 2011). In addition, research on the lived experience of older LGBT people reveals high rates of peer bullying (Fredriksen-Goldsen et al., 2011).

Prevalence rates among youth for witnessing bullying are also informative. A study conducted in one school district that included 75 elementary schools, 20 middle schools, and 14 high schools (15,185 students) found that 70.4% of the students reported they had seen incidents of bullying at school, 62% had witnessed bullying at least two times in the last month, and 41% had witnessed bullying once a week or more (Bradshaw, Sawyer, & O'Brennan, 2007). Furthermore, school employees tended to underestimate the number of students involved in bullying, and those with greater confidence in their ability to address bullying incidents were more likely to actually intervene when bullying occurred (Bradshaw et al., 2007). Likeliness to intervene when bullying takes place is critical because evidence suggests that bystander intervention stops bullying within 10 seconds nearly 60% of the time, as discussed in Chapter 7 (Hawkins, Pepler, & Craig, 2001). This is especially relevant because only 20%–30% of youth who are bullied actually report to someone in authority that they were bullied (Ttofi & Farrington, 2010). These prevalence rates suggest that residents of senior housing communities and participants in communal senior services may provide administrators and service delivery personnel with the most accurate information about the extent of peer bullying occurring in their organizations. The high likelihood that older adults are similarly reluctant to inform anyone of their own bullying experiences means that witness reports may be a primary source for identifying problems. Other chapters elaborate on how to survey resident or consumer populations to determine the extent and range of bullying and antagonistic behaviors that are occurring. The effectiveness of bystander intervention in combination with residents' and consumers' likelihood of witnessing bullying among their peers suggests the importance of training older adults themselves in how to intervene. Chapter 7 outlines such an intervention.

The importance of staff in stopping or defusing bullying situations points to the value of training staff to view bullying as a problem, to recognize bullying, and to have the skills to intervene. Chapter 9 outlines a foundational staff training program to help senior housing and social service staff learn to effectively address bullying and other challenging behaviors among older adults.

Anti-Bullying Interventions for Children and Youth

Research supports that a positive school climate minimizes the occurrence of bullying. For example, the targets of bullying are less likely to choose aggressive responses to defend themselves and more likely to seek support from school staff when they report higher levels of school safety and connectedness (Moon, McCluskey, & Schreck, 2013). The most effective climate improvement programs involve school-wide efforts with multiple components emphasizing the reduction of aggression and bullying across a variety of settings. In accordance with an ecological framework, these programs often include instituting school-wide policies, including parents in trainings and or meetings, and increasing playground supervision (Leff & Waasdorp, 2013). As such, older adults are likely to be less antagonistic in positive living or socialization environments. Chapter 4 outlines a three-level intervention model to create a caring community that is likely to minimize bullying and other challenging relationship behaviors.

Mindfulness and Mindfulness-Based Stress Reduction

One intervention that can aid in the prevention of bullying in schools is the use of mindfulness and mindfulness-based stress reduction (MBSR). This intervention provides students with the tools to respond, rather than simply react, when feeling angry, anxious, or other uncomfortable emotions that can trigger aggressive and bullying behaviors. A primary component of mindfulness is focusing on the breath, which can help regulate the autonomic nervous system (Napoli, Krech, & Holley, 2005). Mindfulness focuses on paying attention to each moment without judgment and then choosing a course of action that is most beneficial (Purcell & Murphy, 2014). In adolescents, the neocortex portion of the brain responsible for critical thinking is not yet fully developed.

Therefore, young people do not have the cognitive ability to effectively handle intense emotions, making them prone to reactive outbursts. Mindfulness skills help adolescents temper emotional responses, which can minimize aggressive actions such as bullying. Among school children, mindfulness training is associated with improved self-esteem, improved mood, lower anxiety, and reduced behavioral problems (Napoli, Krech, & Holley, 2005), all traits connected to less involvement with bullying as either a bully or target.

Research has shown that mindfulness also helps adults to minimize emotional reactivity, thus allowing individuals to avoid letting anger escalate into aggressive behavior. For example, adults who scored higher on measures of mindfulness skills, such as awareness of physical and emotional experiences, not criticizing their feelings and emotional responses, and not impulsively reacting to their feelings and emotional responses, were less likely to respond with anger to difficult situations (Hirano & Yukawa, 2014). Therefore, incorporating mindfulness within senior housing and service organizations may be a practical way to minimize bullying. Chapter 8 details an empathy-based anti-bullying intervention that incorporates mindfulness components.

Summary

This chapter has reviewed two sources of bullying-related research, a small group of studies that focus on challenging behaviors among older adults, and a large group of studies that focus on children and youth. In particular, insights into negative social interactions among younger people offer a unique understanding of bullying behaviors that occur later in life and inform the anti-bullying interventions presented in this book.

CHAPTER 3

Understanding Older People Who Bully and Those Who Are Bullied

Older People Who Bully

As described in Chapter 2, individuals who bully tend to have a strong need to control and dominate others. Some speculate that the adage "once a bully, always a bully" holds true and theorize that older adults who bully also engaged in peer bullying during their youth (Rice, 2014). However, in keeping with the strengths perspective it is vital to acknowledge other factors that may contribute to negative behaviors. The strengths perspective focuses on a person's strengths as a foundation for change, rather than focusing exclusively on challenging behaviors and the need to eliminate them (Saleebey, 2006). It also recognizes that challenging behaviors may be a reaction to the environment and do not solely stem from interpersonal deficits.

First, bullies tend to put others down in order to build themselves up, suggesting low self-esteem may play a role in their social interaction patterns. For example, John, who resides in an independent housing community, would often intimidate peers with his power wheelchair while they were walking in the hallway, threatening to run them over if they did not get out of his way. He especially targeted peers who tended to walk slowly or who used an assistive device. Upon discussing this behavior with a social worker, John confessed that he felt envious and "less than" his fellow residents who could walk because he had been confined to a wheelchair for several years. "Real men go on two legs," he said. This is an example of how negative feelings about one's self can contribute to bullying others who have a desired attribute or skill.

Second, loss is ubiquitous with aging in Western societies, including loss of independence, relationships, income, and valued roles. Such losses are especially salient for those who transition to assisted living, skilled nursing facilities, and other long-term care settings, where losses can extend to one's social identity and sense of belonging. Older adults who find themselves living among strangers and being helped by staff may struggle with defining who they are and how they fit in. Thus, older individuals who bully may be seeking greater control at a time in life when they feel especially powerless, and bullying behaviors may be attempts to regain a sense of equilibrium related to overwhelming changes (Bonifas & Frankel, 2012). Fear of future loss may also be a factor. In Chapter 8, Alyse November shares several stories of people who excluded others from social gatherings as the individuals being excluded experienced functional decline. Subsequent intervention revealed the person doing the excluding was confronting fears of his or her own future decline, which contributed to the relationally aggressive bullying behavior.

Third, the majority of residents in long-term care may never have lived in a communal setting; if they have, it was likely in the remote past, perhaps during their schooling or military service. Shared living requires adjustments regarding territory and personal space, and feelings of jealousy and impatience often arise. The diversity of values, beliefs, and experiences inherent in communities for older adults can magnify such negative reactions (see Chapter 2). Some bullying behaviors related to territoriality, such as exerting control over program viewing with shared televisions, dining room seating arrangements, and the time and attention of staff, may reflect underlying attempts to adjust to communal living by changing public space into private space.

Bonifas and Hector (2013) examined differences between individuals who bully and those who do not in assisted living settings. Among characteristics assessed, which included cognitive status, self-esteem, depressive symptoms, and lifetime incidence of trauma, individuals who bullied others differed from their peers in two areas: cognitive status and exposure to lifetime trauma. There were no differences in terms of self-esteem levels; both groups tended to report moderate levels of self-esteem. As noted in Chapter 2, residents who bullied tended to not have any cognitive impairments, whereas residents not identified as bullies more often did have cognitive impairments. From a practical perspective, in organizations where regular interaction occurs between these two groups, care needs to be taken to monitor social relationship patterns to detect and address bullying behaviors. Chapters 7 and 8 propose strategies to help identify and minimize such dynamics.

Surprisingly, according to Bonifas and Hector (2013), assisted living residents who engaged in bullying reported fewer incidents of lifetime trauma (five) compared to their counterparts who did not bully (eight). Traumatic events were based on the Life Events Checklist (Gray, Litz, Hsu, & Lombardo, 2004) and included items such as natural disasters, transportation accidents, physical assault, war experiences, and life-threatening illnesses or injuries. It is possible that experiencing less adversity across the life course may be related to the lack of empathy noted among bullies in other research studies. Empathy refers to "feeling with" or being able to understand the experience or feelings of another. In Chapter 8, Alyse November helpfully refers to this as "being able to stand in another person's shoes." Individuals who bully may have less insight into how others are feeling and how their behaviors impact others. In other words, when one has experienced painful life events, one develops greater insight into the feelings of others who have endured similar distressful events. When one has not experienced such adversity, it can be difficult to walk in the shoes of people who have. Additional research is needed to determine the validity of this hypothesis, as well as if the nature of lifetime trauma is different for individuals who bully versus those who do not.

Other characteristics common among older people who bully include the following, as identified by helping professionals working on anti-bullying efforts in senior care environments (personal communication, Marsha Frankel, personal communication, March 31, 2013):

- using power and control strategies at the expense of others

- putting others down to build themselves up

- gaining positive reinforcement by making others feel threatened, fearful or hurt, and by fueling conflict between people

- experiencing difficulty tolerating individual differences

For example, David, when asked to explain his tendency of intimidating staff and residents at his senior housing community, replied: "It's fun to make them jump when I start in on them!" David felt an enhanced sense of control and personal power when his behavior toward others rapidly initiated a response.

Individuals who bully also tend to have very few social relationships. However, it is unclear whether those who bully have few social relationships because people do not want to befriend a bully, or because individuals who have few friends and feel they are not well liked may be prone to engage in bullying behaviors. More research is needed to tease out the connection between these two factors.

Senior care providers can ask the following questions of individuals known to engage in bullying behaviors to identify potential underlying needs. Note that these questions do not address bullying behaviors directly; individuals who bully are rarely willing to admit that they engage in such behaviors. Rather, questions focus on identifying difficulties the individual is experiencing that may be contributing to negative social behaviors.

- What has changed for you over the past year or two?

- What has concerned you the most over the past year or two?

- How have your feelings about yourself changed over the past year or two?

- What is most challenging for you about living here [for senior housing] or coming here [for senior centers, adult day centers, etc.]?

- What thoughts do you have about the other people who live here [for senior housing] or come here [for senior centers, adult day centers, etc.]?

- Many people feel less of a sense of being in control as they mature and experience life changes. What kinds of things have been difficult for you to have less control over?

- What gives you a sense of being more in control of things?

A resident's responses can help staff identify potential underlying needs that, if met, could stop bullying behaviors. For example, imagine that Marge is interviewed and gives the following responses:

- What has changed for you over the past year or two?

  Well, I had to move out of my house. I lived there for 50 years. Had the best yard in the neighborhood, can you believe that? People used to come to me for advice on growing everything from zucchini to zinnias. I don't have a garden now; this arthritis keeps me from digging and pruning. Always had me a dog, too, always well behaved. No constant barking like that yip-yap my idiot neighbor has. People used to ask me how to train up their dog like mine.

- What has concerned you the most over the past year or two?

  I don't really like living with all these people; lots of weirdos here. Like that guy down the hall from me. He's a mess: dirty clothes, dirty hair, needs to shave, he stinks to high heaven, too. In my day, both men and women were presentable. There are a lot of young slobs around here. I think this place should be for older people only.

- How have your feelings about yourself changed over the past year or two?

  I am not sure what you mean. I am fine. I don't like my arthritis and the pain and aches it gives me, but I am still me. It's others that are the problem. They aren't interested in gardening here or in training up their dogs right.

- What is most challenging for you about living here?

  That's an easy one! The people! Too many weird ones, talking to themselves, getting in my way, watching stupid TV programs. There's one that all she wants is "The Price is Right," stupidest show ever, especially without Bob Barker. I don't think there is one person with any intelligence here.

- What thoughts do you have about the other people who live here or come here?

  Well, I guess I just told you some of them. There's no one like me here. They don't like the things I like, they don't appreciate what I know. No one wants to hear about why the plants are dying on the patio or how to get that apple tree free from worms.

- Many people feel less of a sense of being in control as they mature and experience life changes. What kinds of things have been difficult for you to have less control over?

    It's really hard not to have my own place. I know I have my own room, but it's not my place. I can't decorate it the way I want. There's no room for a garden. My window doesn't even look out onto a tree or a flower, not even a weed. And wherever I go, there's these idiot people that live here. There is really no one I like. I try to tell them what to do so they can be better, be a bit more intelligent and interesting, but it does no good. People used to listen to me, but they don't now, no matter how hard I yell.

- What gives you a sense of being more in control of things?

    I like telling people about things and having them appreciate what I tell them. I like people asking me about stuff and giving advice. These bozos here don't want to know anything.

It is important to first recognize that these responses are shorter than they would likely be in reality and that Marge is more forthcoming with her answers than an actual bully might be. A positive, trusting relationship would be needed between Marge and the interviewer for her to openly express her feelings, and questions might need to be asked over a period of time. In addition, a nonjudgmental attitude on the part of the interviewer is imperative.

Marge's pattern of responses suggests that she is having a hard time adjusting to not being the valued advice giver in her neighborhood. She appears to feel unappreciated by and disconnected from her peers; she believes that they are very different from her and beneath her in many respects. She feels in control when she has information to share and appears to be trying to gain a sense of control by bossing others around and yelling at them, possibly even by being overly critical. An intervention plan to minimize the likelihood that Marge will engage in bullying behaviors might focus on arranging opportunities for her to give advice in more healthy and productive ways, perhaps by guiding staff in efforts to care for the plants and trees on the patio or by having Marge write a how-to manual for training dogs that could be featured in the gift shop. Similarly, a window box might be installed outside of her room to allow gardening activity with adaptive tools to accommodate her arthritis. Enhancing Marge's general satisfaction in life will result in less antagonistic behavior toward her peers. In addition, she will have less time on her hands to focus on negativity. Of course, such an individual approach to thwarting bullying behaviors is not the only solution. For readers who may be interested in looking at bullying at an organizational rather than individual level, Chapter 7 includes a survey instrument to assess the extent of bullying in a senior living setting.

Older People Who Are Bullied

In contrast to people who bully, the targets of bullying often have passive social interaction styles that create vulnerability to bullies' efforts to dominate them (Batsche & Knoff, 1994). They may have trouble defending themselves and may be unsure of how to effectively respond to being targeted (Olweus, 1993). For example, a senior housing resident in Kansas City reported that the bullying behaviors of another resident hindered her from spending time with her sister. This distressed her so much that she took an overdose of prescription medication, in part because "she didn't know how to respond to the bully" (Rice, 2014, p. 1).

It is interesting to note that not all individuals who were exposed to the same challenging encounters were as negatively affected by their experiences. As mentioned earlier, to account for these differences in bullying-related emotional distress, Bonifas and Hector (2013) assessed the cognitive status, depressive symptoms, self-esteem, and lifetime exposure to trauma of individuals who were targeted. Findings revealed that the residents who were most upset by being bullied had higher rates of depressive symptoms and lower self-esteem (Bonifas & Kramer, 2012). In addition, as identified by similarities in their social histories, they were more likely to have been bullied by their peers as children (Bonifas, 2011). It is possible that depressive symptoms and low self-esteem cause some older individuals to react more strongly to bullying situations.

Among older individuals who exhibit resilience in response to bullying, various coping strategies may help to minimize negative consequences, including the following:

- Avoid contact with the individual.

- Walk away from negative encounters.

- Engage in positive self-talk.

- "Bite your tongue."

- Pursue individual activities.

- Tune out the behavior.

- Strive to see the other person's point of view.

- Offer alternatives to challenging behaviors.

- Work to calm others down.

- Spend time with pets.

- Nurture relationships with supportive individuals.

Bullying Can Create an Overwhelming Sense of Helplessness

Targets of bullying often experience a sense of powerlessness and anxiety because incidents are unpredictable. These feelings are magnified due to the difficulties they face in preventing incidents and in removing themselves from bullying situations (personal communication, Marsha Frankel, March 30, 2012). The June 2012 "bullies on the bus" incident in which 68-year-old Karen Klein was subjected to verbal tormenting while performing her bus monitor duties illustrates such helplessness. Although the bullies were children rather than peers of her age group, the characteristics of the incident offer insight into the dynamics of a bullying experience can create feelings of helplessness. In interviews, Ms. Klein describes positioning herself on the bus in the second to last seat, which inadvertently allowed the boys to surround her. This seating arrangement seemed to contribute to their power in the situation. Although Ms. Klein was an adult and an intended authority figure on the bus, she was unable to extricate herself from the situation, even when the boys' comments drove her to tears. If she had felt some personal power in the situation, she might have gotten up and moved to a seat closer to the bus driver where she could still monitor the children but have the protection of another adult nearby. This example is in no way meant to blame Ms. Klein, but rather to illustrate how the usurpation of one's power can result in helplessness and an inability to act.

As another example of helplessness and the inability to take action, a woman in an independent senior housing community found it distressing to be continually exposed to her peers' derogatory comments toward supportive services staff working in the building, individuals she found to be helpful and who were important to her life. She felt her peers' negative comments were a personal criticism because she liked and appreciated the staff. To minimize distress, she elected to avoid all contact with these peers, which meant more time spent alone when she would rather have been engaged in community activities. Although she reported feeling upset by her peers' negative comments, she did not even think of banding together with other residents who also appreciated the supportive services staff (Bonifas, 2011).

Types of Bullying
Targets Among Older Adults

According to Olweus (1993), there are two types of bullying targets—passive and provocative. Passive targets tend to show a lot of emotion, are often anxious, and typically do not read social cues well. People who interact with them may perceive them as shy and insecure. They do not initiate bullying or challenging interactions, but instead passively engage in behaviors that disturb others. Among older adults, such targets may have early-stage dementia, a developmental disability, or a mental health condition (Bonifas & Frankel, 2012). A resident in assisted living describes the difficulty of living with an individual who was a passive target of bullying: "You can't get away from that certain person, it's hard, it's hard. She won't change. She does this to everybody, every day. Just aggravates the [expletive] out of me." The referenced individual anxiously and repeatedly recited *The Lord's Prayer* during congregate meals, not recognizing that others did not wish to hear it, and was often the subject of much ridicule and outright animosity. This person is a passive target of bullying because although she does not interact or engage with others by displaying annoying or disruptive behaviors, she unwittingly antagonizes others just the same.

Provocative targets can be annoying or irritating to others, such as by intruding into their personal space. They are often perceived as quick-tempered, and their behaviors that frustrate others may unintentionally invite bullying behaviors. Among older adults, such individuals may have more severe cognitive impairments or a mental health condition. For example, an assisted living resident with schizophrenia who really liked pizza often persisted on the topic of his favorite meal, loudly and repeatedly requesting pizza orders in public areas of the building. Other residents found this behavior highly annoying and would yell at him to shut up, shout obscenities, and ridicule him with taunts of "pizza-pizza-pizza man" (Bonifas, 2011).

Differences Can Create Vulnerability for Being Bullied

As mentioned earlier in the chapter, older adults who are perceived as different from the majority of residents in senior housing settings may become the targets of bullying behaviors because bullies have difficulty tolerating individual differences. People who have just moved in are among those most at risk, as are those with newly acquired and readily apparent functional limitations. Rice (2014) detailed the experience of an 84-year-old senior housing resident who faced bullying after she began using a wheelchair following a stroke. Initially, only one person was involved in verbally bullying the woman, telling her that her wheelchair was too wide, that she could not care for herself properly, and that she smelled bad. But then others engaged in relational aggression and shunned the woman.

Minority status based on race, ethnicity, religious background, or perceived sexual orientation can also single out individuals for bullying. For instance, one assisted living resident reported that, "[because of my African American race], many people assume I am up to something . . . I [was] wrongfully accused of being with someone else's girlfriend and [was] yelled at in the hallway [by another resident]" (Bonifas, 2011). Another example occurred in a conversational English class for older adults. A small group of well-educated women from Russia were relationally aggressive toward a less-educated newcomer from China. They rolled their eyes whenever she would speak and made snide comments about her in Russian (Bonifas & Frankel, 2012). Anecdotal reports also indicate that older adults may be teased, mocked, or ridiculed or excluded from joining group activities for speaking with a foreign accent or with limited proficiency in English (Marsha Frankel, personal communication, March 30, 2012).

Older adults are also bullied on the basis of their sexuality. Men may have their heterosexuality openly questioned in a demeaning way, and bullies may spread rumors about women's alleged promiscuity (Bonifas, 2011). Glen, an older gay man who participated in Bonifas and Kramer's (2011) study of negative social relationships in assisted living, noted that other residents viewed homosexuality with "a lot of personal hate and fear. . . . It's a generational thing . . . younger people accept gay people and lesbians; people my age don't" (Bonifas, 2011). Exposure to pervasive homophobia took its toll on Glen. For example, several heterosexual men in the residential facility where Glen lived reported being *accused* of being gay. These accusations were viewed as highly insulting and the topic of angry debate in communal areas. Glen described what it was like to regularly hear the outrage of peers who felt the ultimate insult was an insinuation that they were like him. "I got down, really down . . . it was really, really unfair to say something like that to be mean, it was awful" (Bonifas, 2011).

Warning Signs that an Individual Is Being Bullied

Although some older adults will report incidents of bullying to senior housing or senior center staff, others fear peer reprisal and will not. Unfortunately, staff members may not witness bullying among their residents because it often takes the form of relational aggression. Organizational personnel should err on the side of caution and assume that bullying is occurring, even if challenging interactions are not immediately apparent. Remember that children on the playground do not usually torment one another when the principal is watching. There are, however, some warning signs, including the following, that indicate someone may be the target of bullying:

- Person avoids specific areas of the residence or senior center or certain activities of interest.

- Person takes long, circuitous routes to get to and from communal facility areas.

- Person voices vague complaints about peers, such as "They don't like me" or "They won't let me."

- A new resident or center participant reports feeling unwelcomed or having difficulty fitting in or making friends.

- Multiple residents complain about a specific resident or group of residents.

- Staff members express discomfort interacting with a specific resident or center participant.

It is important to recognize that vulnerable targets of bullying may present in an angry manner, but they rarely present in a powerful manner. Indeed, they may be too intimidated to report having been targeted at all. When an individual claims in a loud, intimidating, boisterous manner that he or she is being bullied, usually this person is actually the bully and is experiencing pushback from peers trying to set limits on his or her behavior. Sometimes retaliatory bullying occurs when peers target the initial bully in an attempt to control his or her challenging behaviors.

Summary

This chapter reviewed the common characteristics of older people who bully others and how these traits can inform approaches to minimize bullying behaviors. In addition, this chapter discussed strategies for evaluating the potential underlying needs of individuals who engage in bullying, the characteristics of those who tend to be targeted by bullies, associated implications for intervention, and warning signs that can alert care providers that bullying may be occurring in their community. Chapter 4 begins the section on general approaches to address bullying among older adults.

PART II

General Interventions to Address Bullying Among Older Adults

CHAPTER 4

A Framework for
Anti-Bullying Interventions

Interventions to address bullying among older adults must consider what older adults themselves have to say about potentially effective strategies, especially given that they may witness bullying incidents more often than staff members do. Assisted living residents offered the following suggestions for how senior living organizations can decrease bullying and other problematic social behaviors (Bonifas, 2011):

- *Conduct onsite anger management classes.* Older adults surveyed felt that many problematic interactions between residents stemmed from difficulties people had controlling their feelings of anger. By offering constructive ways for residents to manage anger and channel intense emotions, the general milieu of the organizational environment would improve.

- *Strive to set limits for people who bully or "pick on" others.* Administrative staff should approach those who bully others, inform them that their behavior is not acceptable, and request that they cease and desist. Staff should then provide these people with suggestions for acceptable behaviors. For example, the first part of setting limits might be telling a resident that she may not save seats during leisure activities because doing so excludes others. The second part might involve reminding her that she and her friends are welcome to enter at the same time and will be helped to find seats together.

- *Work collaboratively with residents to minimize the occurrence of bullying behaviors and other negative social interactions.* Regular meetings to promote communication about the relationship challenges associated with communal living and to identify potential resolutions to those challenges could prevent episodes of bullying. Such meetings might take the form of a monthly resident council group through which any resident could submit concerns related to negative social interactions for council discussion and could do so anonymously, if preferred. The group could then discuss what had happened and, together with organizational leadership, investigate further, determine a course of action, and implement necessary interventions.

- *Develop written policy and procedure statements to guide acceptable behaviors among residents.* These rules could serve as a foundation to help enforce civil social interactions and inform residents about behaviors that are not permitted, with the understanding that some individuals may not inherently know what behaviors are inappropriate.

A Three-Tier Intervention Model

Preventing and minimizing bullying requires multiple interventions focused on each component of the bullying equation: the organization, the bullies, and the targets of bullying. Of these three, organizational-level intervention is the most crucial. When bullying is addressed at the organizational level, the underlying needs of individuals who bully are often met and the difficulties of those who are prone to bullying are often minimized, such that less intervention is needed at these two levels. The value of organizational-level intervention can be difficult for senior living and senior care providers to acknowledge because their expectation is that only the bully needs to change. However, the most positive outcomes are achieved by using a combined set of approaches that combat bullying behaviors from several angles.

Organizational Interventions

In approaching bullying from an organizational level, the focus is on preventing its occurrence. The goal is to create a caring and empathetic community along with an organizational culture that does not tolerate bullying. *Caring* refers to feeling and exhibiting concern for others; *empathetic* refers to the capacity to recognize and share another's feelings. Accomplishing this requires that both older adults and staff members work together as partners in managing problematic social interactions. Therefore, intervention efforts should not focus exclusively on residents or participants alone, but should also include staff members. Elaine Bourne explains the value of using a combined approach based on her training sessions for managing conflict among older adults. "We have found . . . in the facilities [where] staff participated [in the training] . . . there was actually [a greater reduction in interpersonal] conflicts (personal communication, March 30, 2014).

Creating Caring Communities

Caring and empathetic communities first strive to establish an organizational culture that does not foster or tolerate bullying. In an environment that promotes empathy, there is an atmosphere of respect and trust. Residents and staff are held accountable for their behaviors, which sets the stage for people being willing to defend themselves and others, a key factor in eliminating bullying behaviors. An attitude of caring and empathy must be embraced by the entire organization; residents, staff, and management must make a commitment to promote and live by the tenets of equality and respect for all members of the community. Some senior centers ask attendees to sign a code of conduct attesting that they will treat all participants with respect and will refrain from subjecting them to "yelling, obscene language, and other verbal abuse" (Creno, 2010). This philosophy, while a good start, needs to extend to include staff members and management as well.

Decreasing Bullying by Increasing Positive Behaviors

Incorporating strategies that increase caring and empathetic behaviors is also critical in decreasing bullying episodes. As positive behaviors increase, problematic interactions will naturally diminish. Interventions can be fairly simple and might include the following:

- Acknowledge members of the community who go out of their way to welcome new residents or participants or anyone who is perceived as different.

- Institute a "Caring Squad" whose job is to notice and reward acts of kindness.

- Nominate "Empathy Leaders" each month to recognize residents and staff who have been especially compassionate.

Such approaches send the message throughout the community that caring and empathy are effective ways to achieve recognition, which is important for bullies who may seek attention through negative behavior. (See Chapter 7 for a complete overview of a three-step intervention designed to increase positive interactions in long-term care settings.)

Examples of Organizational Interventions

Ongoing training and communication-building opportunities to help both residents and staff effectively address bullying behaviors are vital components of anti-bullying efforts. Three organizational-level interventions that senior care professionals across the country have found helpful to equip older adults and care providers with the skills and knowledge necessary to decrease bullying and to bolster caring and empathy include modified peace learning circles, civility training, and bystander intervention training.

Modified Peace Learning Circles

In striving to create a more caring community, one assisted living facility started a resident council group that met regularly to discuss and resolve problematic issues within the community. The group developed a training workshop designed to sensitize residents to bullying behaviors and build their skill set for intervening when they observed inappropriate peer interactions (Michelle James, personal communication, April 6, 2012). Based on a teaching module developed by *Peace Learning Circles, Incorporated,* for use among school children, the residents devised a workshop led by a psychology intern that featured several components (visit http://www.peacelearningcircles.com/). First, workshop leaders reviewed various types of problematic behaviors and provided attendees with opportunities to add examples from their own experiences. Then, they featured a humorous skit that demonstrated the power that one individual has to create a negative environment, followed by a discussion of how, alternatively, just one individual can create a positive environment. They then presented several simple strategies to defuse tension, such as calling attention to stress ("Looks like things are getting a little hot between you two"); using humor ("Whoa, settle down you two prize fighters"); and distraction with redirection ("How about you two agree to disagree and let's go get some hot coffee"). Participants then engaged in brief role-play scenarios to practice using these intervention strategies when interactions between peers started to intensify. (See Figure 4.1 at the end of this chapter for instructions for setting up a modified peace learning circle.)

Although the anti-bullying workshop went well, the resident council group was disappointed with its implementation because the people whom they felt really needed the intervention did not attend, and some people who did attend had trouble paying attention for the entire session. Rather than becoming discouraged, the resident council decided to incorporate additional approaches that were better tailored to the range of interests and ability levels within the community. First, they met with the facility chaplain to devise a plan to incorporate the workshop's positive teachings into the weekly religious service, an event attended by the majority of residents. Then they decided to feature positive messages about caring and empathy on the monthly activity calendar that most residents consulted daily. Example positive messages included "Do unto others as you would have done unto you"; "Kindness never goes out of style"; "Everyone belongs; everyone has a place"; and "If you can't say anything nice, don't say anything at all."

Civility Training

Diana Benson, Resident Services Coordinator for a senior housing community in Ohio, shared her intervention to create and maintain a bully-free living environment in her organization. Based on

Forni's (2002), *Choosing Civility,* and Speak Your Peace: The Civility Project, of the Duluth Superior Area Community Foundation in Minnesota, Ms. Benson encouraged residents to practice the following nine tools of civility:

1. Pay attention

2. Listen

3. Be inclusive

4. Avoid gossip

5. Show respect

6. Be agreeable

7. Apologize

8. Give constructive criticism

9. Take responsibility

The intervention began with a 9-week warm-up period to pique residents' interest in the program. Words associated with civility, such as *kindness, respect, dignity, compassion, loyalty, forgiveness, understanding, listening,* and *character,* appeared on community bulletin boards and elevator walls without any explanation. Of course, these mysterious words contributed to considerable speculation among community residents. Ms. Benson took great care not to reveal any of her plans when residents approached her with questions, but just said, "You'll see," which made everyone all the more curious. At week 10, all nine slogans as well as an invitation to join the Civility Project were posted together.

The invitation was accompanied by a brief article in the housing community's newsletter that encouraged residents to attend a special presentation on civility a few days later. The presentation emphasized the nine tools of civility and promoted discussion about how to improve relationships within the community as well as specific strategies for how to treat one another with greater respect. For example, participants learned about the importance of honoring other people and their opinions during disagreements, purposely looking for opportunities to agree with others, and sticking to the issues at hand during disputes rather than resorting to personal attacks. At the close of the presentation, residents signed a Civility Pledge (see Figure 4.2, end of chapter) and a Civility Resolution (see Figure 4.3, end of chapter), and were given *Speak Your Peace* cards highlighting the nine civility tools. Readers are encouraged to download their own copies of these materials from http://www.dsaspeakyourpeace.org/free_stuff.html.

Ms. Benson indicated that although not all residents attended the civility presentation, those who did shared the information with their neighbors, and additional residents came to her to get their own *Speak Your Peace* cards. She noted that over time gossiping and rumor-spreading were much less rampant after the intervention. Furthermore, overall morale improved and residents voiced fewer complaints about the negative behaviors of other residents. Community members were also motivated to form a Neighbor-to-Neighbor program that recruited volunteers to visit socially isolated residents, welcome new residents and help them get acquainted with others, and encourage socialization and involvement in group activities. Residents also established a barter system for completing instrumental tasks, such as mending and shopping.

Bystander Intervention Training

Marsha Frankel and Kathy Burnes of Jewish Family & Children's Services of Greater Boston have developed a training program to help older adults take action to reduce social bullying that occurs in their housing communities. Building on the idea that most bullying occurs in the presence of peer witnesses, the 60- to 75-minute training aims to enable older adults to understand what social bullying is, differentiate it from everyday negative behaviors, and learn steps they can personally take to minimize bullying.

The training intervention has three components: (1) an overview of bullying among older adults, (2) a discussion of the cycle of bullying and the role of bystanders in prevention, and (3) skills to thwart bullying. The overview engages participants by asking them to reflect on the question "What do you think of when you hear the term *bullying*?" Facilitators then formally define *bullying*, detail the nature of bullying among older adults, including the characteristics of bullies and targets, and describe how bullying impacts older adults and the communities in which they live. Emphasizing how both bystanders and targets can intervene to disrupt the cycle, presenters then explain the cycle of bullying (Alcon, Burnes, & Frankel, 2014):

1. Bully targets person or persons.

2. Supporters and followers participate in the bullying.

3. Target and onlookers do not intervene.

4. Bully is empowered to continue his or her behavior.

5. Onlookers do not intervene.

6. Cycle of bullying continues to repeat.

During the final component of the training, participants learn three effective options for responding to bullying: (1) defending the target, (2) challenging the bully's behavior, and (3) redirecting or diverting the bullying behavior. Significant focus is given to how to stand up to people who bully by understanding that it is the bully who has the problem, looking the bully in the eye, responding calmly with self-assurance to bullying behaviors, and then walking away (Alcon et al., 2014, p. 17). Facilitators demonstrate skills using brief skits, and then participants practice the new skills in simple role-play scenarios. Example situations include when someone is excluded from a group activity or when someone inappropriately blocks access to seating during communal meals. Interested readers are encouraged to contact the training developers for a copy of the how-to manual through Jewish Family & Children's Services of Greater Boston at http://www.jfcsboston.org. An alternative detailed bystander intervention program is presented in chapter 7.

It is important to understand that developing a caring community is a process, and organizational change is slow; noticeable improvements take time. For instance, after beginning a community culture change effort, staff in one assisted living facility reported that it was several months before residents began to express greater value of others' perspectives (Dr. Jay Hedgpeth, personal communication, June 07, 2012).

Determining the Most Problematic Behaviors and Their Occurrence Rates

Assessing what type of bullying behaviors and other problematic behaviors are most common and how often they occur is a valuable initial step in planning organizational interventions. The questionnaire and instructions presented in Figure 4.4 at the end of the chapter can be used as a tool for conducting such an assessment. Senior care providers can administer the questionnaire to residents, and results can help to guide effective interventions. The first 10 questions are based on the Problematic Social Relationships Questionnaire developed by Trompetter, Scholte, & Westerhof (2011). The remaining 10 questions were developed by the author (Bonifas, 2014) in consultation with a convenience sample of senior housing coordinators across the country who were experiencing bullying among residents in their housing communities. Residents can submit the questionnaire anonymously (e.g., by depositing it in a large ballot box) or through an interview with a staff member or volunteer. Chapter 7 provides useful suggestions for which font sizes are necessary for questionnaires to be in senior environments and other helpful strategies from administration personnel. Chapter 7 also includes another questionnaire that helps pinpoint where and when bullying behaviors and problematic social interactions occur, which can be used to support a more advanced assessment of what is going on when organizational leaders are ready to tailor interventions to specific challenging situations within their facilities.

Analyzing the Questionnaire Results and Using the Findings

After collecting questionnaires from as many residents as possible, responses can be analyzed to determine patterns of bullying behaviors across the senior living community. For example, responses can be tracked and sorted using software such Microsoft Excel, with each survey respondent representing a row of data and the categories representing each of the 20 questions.

Table 4.1.   Sample spreadsheet reflecting partial entries for five participants

	Question 1	Question 2	Question 3	Question 4	Question 5
Participant 1	1	2	2	3	0
Participant 2	0	1	2	1	0
Participant 3	2	0	3	0	1
Participant 4	0	3	3	0	0
Participant 5	1	2	0	1	0
Average of responses	4/5	8/5	10/5	5/5	1/5

Respondents' answers would be entered as numbers in each cell as follows (see Table 4.1):

4 = Several times per day

3 = Several times per week

2 = Several times per month

1 = Every few months

0 = Never

Alternatively, the number of responses in each category for each question can be determined with a calculator.

The goal of analysis is to determine the most common type of problematic behaviors and how frequently they occur. This can be accomplished in two different ways. The easiest way is to calculate an average score for each question. This is done by adding the numbers representing residents' answers for each question and dividing each of the 20 totals by the number of residents who completed the questionnaire. In Table 4.2, results indicate residents experience gossiping and rumor spreading anywhere from several times per month to every few months.

The largest averages represent the most frequent types of bullying or problematic behaviors that the residents who responded to the questionnaire are experiencing. Efforts to minimize bullying in the facility should target those behaviors. Of course,

Table 4.2. Average number of bullying behaviors from the first five questions on the bullying questionnaire for five participants

Question	Average Response
1. Another resident/participant has ignored you on purpose.	4/5 = 0.8
2. Another resident/participant has spread rumors and gossip about you.	8/5 = 1.6
3. Another resident/participant has repeatedly teased you in a hurtful way.	10/5 = 2.0
4. Another resident/participant has made fun of you behind your back.	5/5 = 1.0
5. Another resident/participant has refused to sit at your table on purpose because he or she wishes to avoid you.	1/5 = 0.2

when using the questionnaire in an actual facility, intervention decision making would be based on results from all 20 questions and involve a greater number of residents.

An alternative method that is more complicated, but generates more specific results, is to calculate the percentage of residents who selected each of the five responses for all 20 questions. Rather than adding each resident's actual responses for a question, the number of residents selecting each response category is calculated and then divided by the number of residents who completed the questionnaire, which is then multiplied by 100. For example, using the partial Microsoft Excel table, for question 1, two tenants selected 1 (every few months), one tenant selected 2 (several times per month), and two tenants selected 0 (never). No tenants selected 3 (several times per week) or 4 (several times per day). Dividing each number by the total number of individuals who completed the survey and multiplying the results by 100 yields the following percentages:

several times per day = 0%

several times per week = 0%

several times per month = 40% (2 divided by 5 = 0.4 x 100 = 40)

every few months = 20% (1 divided by 5 = 0.2 x 100 = 20)

never = 40%

Complete results for all five respondents for the first five questions are presented Table 4.3. As with the calculating averages example, when using the questionnaire in an actual facility, results would be calculated for all 20 questions.

These partial results indicate that the most common behaviors are gossiping and rumor spreading as well as hurtful teasing, with 80% of tenants experiencing these behaviors at least every few months. Twenty percent of tenants are experiencing gossiping and rumor spreading several times per week, and 40% several times per month. Hurtful teasing has occurred for 40% of tenants several times per month and another 40% at least every few months. While being made fun of is not as common as gossiping and rumor spreading or hurtful teasing, it is noteworthy that 40% of tenants still experience this behavior several times per week.

The questionnaire can also be administered 3–6 weeks post-intervention to evaluate the impact of efforts to address bullying. If the interventions are having a positive impact, survey results would demonstrate a decrease in the frequency of bullying behaviors. Note that evaluating the impact of an intervention may be more easily depicted for staff members through percentages. For example, it is more meaningful to explain that before bullying interventions were implemented, 40% of tenants experienced a given behavior several times a week, whereas after the interventions were implemented, only 10% experienced the behavior. Alternately, explaining that average scores dropped from 2.0 to 0.5 on a measurement instrument may not hold as much meaning.

Anti-Bullying Policies and Procedures

Senior housing residents and senior center participants need clear guidance on the types of behaviors that are not acceptable in their communities. (See Figure 4.5 at the end of the chapter for an example of a policy statement.) Such guidelines are necessary to clarify what behaviors should not be displayed, and to allow enforcement of rules governing behaviors. When staff and community leaders use a written document to support their enforcement efforts, the process is less onerous. A written document demonstrates that limit-setting and sanctions are clearly not personal and are grounded in rules that apply to all community members. Accordingly, in developing anti-bullying policy and procedure statements, it is effective to involve residents or

Table 4.3. Sample response percentages from the first five questions of the bullying questionnaire (Figure 4.3) for five participants

Questions	Number (#) and percentage (%) of tenants experiencing each bullying behavior											
	Several times per day		Several times per week		Several times per month		Every few months		Never	
	#	%	#	%	#	%	#	%	#	%
1. Another resident/participant has ignored you on purpose.	0	0	0	0	1	20	2	40	2	40
2. Another resident/participant has spread rumors and gossip about you.	0	0	1	20	2	40	1	20	1	20
3. Another resident/participant has repeatedly teased you in a hurtful way.	0	0	0	0	2	40	2	40	1	20
4. Another resident/participant has made fun of you behind your back.	0	0	2	40	0	0	1	20	2	40
5. Another resident/participant has refused to sit at your table on purpose because he or she wishes to avoid you.	0	0	1	20	0	0	0	0	4	80

participants in the process by involving them in planning meetings, voting on what policies are the most important to them, or appointing an advisory council to review documents and make recommendations to strengthen draft statements. Involving residents in decision-making ensures that their values regarding social relationships and interaction patterns are reflected and creates a sense of buy-in. In addition, collaborative construction guarantees that those behaviors that residents find the most challenging are included. Sometimes the social interaction scenarios that are challenging to management and staff do not affect residents or participants most negatively. The following questions can be used to shape the process of writing the guidelines:

1. What peer behaviors and social interaction styles are the most challenging in your organization?

2. What peer behaviors and social interaction styles do residents or participants want help in managing?

3. How will behavior and interpersonal interactions outside the established guidelines be identified and reported?

4. How will you create psychological safety for individuals who report bullying behaviors, both residents and staff members?

5. How will you document or keep record of incidents and responses?

6. How will you enforce guidelines for resident behaviors and interpersonal interactions? Who will be responsible for enforcement?

7. How will you create psychological and physical safety for individuals responsible for enforcement?

8. What will be the timeline for responding to reports about behaviors and interpersonal interactions outside the guidelines?

9. What sanctions will resident or participants face when they act outside the guidelines?

10. How will you manage serious infringements of others' rights?

11. Who should help your organization with complex situations?

12. What training do residents or participants and staff need to comply with and enforce the policy and procedures effectively?

Summary

This chapter outlined a three-tier framework to minimize bullying behaviors that focuses interventions at the organization level as well as on individuals who bully and the target of bullying. Using a multi-level approach maximizes the impact of interventions so that bullying behaviors and their associated outcomes are minimized as much as possible. The chapter also reviewed promising anti-bullying strategies to bolster caring and empathy among members of the senior housing community that include modified peace learning circles, civility training, and bystander intervention training. The chapter also presented a needs assessment instrument to help detect the range and extent of bullying in an organization and discussed the importance of developing anti-bullying policies and procedures to share with senior housing residents, senior center participants, and staff. Chapter 5 reviews foundational interventions to address bullying behaviors directly with those who bully.

Modified Peace Learning Circle

Purpose of the Activity
The purpose of this activity is to introduce members of our assisted living community to strategies that create peace when people we live with are in observable conflict.

Learning Objectives
Upon completion of this activity, community members will:

1. Understand that it takes only one person to make or break peace.
2. Grasp the importance of inclusion.
3. Recognize negative social behaviors.
4. Draw attention to negative social behavior without embarrassing others.

Time Required: 45 minutes

Materials needed: White board or flip chart

Procedure: Two facilitators are needed. Participants are invited to sit in a circle or around a table.

Part 1. Making Peace
Engage participants in a discussion about problematic social interactions. First, share a few examples of common problematic interactions that tend to occur in the building, such as name-calling, gossiping, excluding people from groups, or making fun of people. Then invite participants to share social interactions that bother them.

Ask: What do other people who live here do or say to you that makes you feel uncomfortable, upset, or angry?

Introduce the concept of peace.

Say: Peace is when people do or say things that make us feel comfortable, calm, and happy.

Engage participants in a discussion of what makes peace and what breaks peace.

Figure 4.1. Instructions for a modified peace learning circle *(continued)*

Ask: How many people does it take to make peace?

Acknowledge each answer, but do not say whether the answer is right or wrong.

Ask: "How many people does it take to break peace?"

Acknowledge each answer, but do not say whether the answer is right or wrong.

Stage a demonstration of how easy it is to break peace:

One facilitator steps away from the group saying he or she has to get something, then comes back in and angrily yells at the other facilitator, "I told you to leave the handouts on my desk! Why don't you ever do what you are told?"

This person leaves again and comes back behaving normally.

Ask: How did you feel when I came back angry?

Encourage participants to share their reactions. Explain that it takes only one person to make or break peace. Stress that each of us can have either a positive or negative impact on others.

Say: Sometimes just drawing attention to a negative behavior can diffuse it. For example, saying, "Looks like you're feeling upset" can help calm someone who is creating a negative social interaction.

Ask: What other ways can we make peace when negative social interactions occur?

Write participants' suggestions on the white board or flip chart. Acknowledge participants' ideas.

Part 2. Making Peace with Negative Behaviors

Say: Let's spend a little more time talking about negative social interactions.

Write three negative social behaviors on the white board or flip chart. For example:

- Making negative comments about someone's hairstyle
- Teasing someone about his or her speech impediment
- Telling someone he or she doesn't belong

Figure 4.1. Instructions for a modified peace learning circle *(continued)*

Ask: What other negative social behaviors happen among us that should be included on this list?

Add suggestions to the list until there are 10 or so.

Say: Remember it takes one person to break peace, but one person can make peace.

Ask: What should we do to make peace if we see one of these social interactions happening in our building?

Write participants' suggestions on the white board or flip chart. Acknowledge participants' ideas.

Say: Here are some additional ways we can make peace. For example, we can call attention to stress levels by saying: "It looks like things are getting a little hot between you two"; by using humor: "Whoa, settle down you two prize fighters"; or by trying to distract those involved: "How about you two agree to disagree and let's go get some hot coffee." Let's practice using these strategies along with the ones you have suggested.

Have everyone form groups of three. Give each group the following scenarios, and have them practice for 10 minutes using the various strategies. Roles should rotate so each member of the group has an opportunity to practice making peace with a few different approaches from the list.

Scenario 1: One tenant refuses to allow another tenant to join in a card game.

Scenario 2: One resident makes fun of another tenant's accent.

Scenario 3: One resident shares some gossip about another tenant who flirted with someone's spouse.

Ask: How did it feel making peace? How confident do you feel about using these techniques in real life?

Encourage the participants to try making peace at least once during the upcoming week and thank them for participating in the activity.

Figure 4.1. Instructions for a modified peace learning circle

Civility Pledge

In all of my daily interactions I pledge to do my best to:

View everyone in positive terms

Work on building common language

Build strong relationships of trust

Remember our shared humanity

Look both inside and outside for guidance

Through this pledge I acknowledge that:

Everyone has the right and responsibility

to improve his or her community,

and if we all work together in a well-planned way

to address the factors that impact all of our lives,

we can make a difference for all residents.

As members of society, we are *all* resources

and agents of change.

Signature: _____

Date: _____

Figure 4.2. Civility Pledge (Newman & Roberts, 2001)

Civility Resolution

WHEREAS, the residents of [insert facility/building name] place a high value on respect and civility in their lives and they understand that these characteristics are essential to any health community, and

WHEREAS, we, the residents, support opportunities for civil discourse and discussion in our community.

WHEREAS, an uncivil and disrespectful atmosphere can have a damaging effect on the residents themselves.

NOW THEREFORE BE IT RESOLVED by the residents of [insert facility/building name] to recognize the nine tenets of civility, which if followed will provide increased opportunities for civil discourse in order to find positive resolutions to the issues that face our community. These tools include the following:

1. Pay attention
2. Listen
3. Be inclusive
4. Avoid gossip
5. Show respect
6. Be agreeable
7. Apologize
8. Give constructive criticism
9. Take responsibility

Resident signatures: _____

_____

_____

_____

Figure 4.3. Civility Resolution (Duluth Superior Area Community Foundation, n.d.)

Bullying Questionnaire

Questions: Considering your experiences of the past year or since moving in/starting to participate in activities. How often have the following situations happened to you?

	Several times per day	Several times per week	Several times per month	Every few months	Never
1. Another resident/participant has ignored you on purpose.	4	3	2	1	0
2. Another resident/participant has spread rumors and gossip about you.	4	3	2	1	0
3. Another resident/participant has repeatedly teased you in a hurtful way.	4	3	2	1	0
4. Another resident/participant has made fun of you behind your back.	4	3	2	1	0
5. Another resident/participant has refused to sit at your table on purpose because he or she wishes to avoid you.	4	3	2	1	0
6. Another resident/participant has made efforts to motivate others to dislike you or to stop having contact with you.	4	3	2	1	0

Figure 4.4. Bullying Questionnaire (Questions 1–10 based on Trompetter, Scholte, & Westerhof [2011]; Questions 11–20 based on Bonifas [2014].) *(Continued)*

From Trompetter, H., Scholte, R., & Westerhof, G. (2011). Resident-to-resident relational aggression and subjective well-being in assisted living facilities. *Aging and Mental Health, 15*, 59–67.
Bonifas, R. P. (January, 2014). Relational aggression in assisted living facilities: Insights into an under-recognized phenomenon. Paper presentation at the 18th Annual Conference of the Society for Social Work Research, San Antonio, Texas.
Appearing in *Bullying Among Older Adults: How to Recognize and Address an Unseen Epidemic*, by Robin P. Bonifas.

7. Another resident/participant has asked you in an unfriendly manner why you live in the building/attend the center.	4	3	2	1	0
8. Another resident/participant has not allowed you to join a group of residents, even if you treat him or her in a friendly way.	4	3	2	1	0
9. Another resident/participant has excluded you from group activities (such as playing cards).	4	3	2	1	0
10. Another resident/participant has criticized you behind your back.	4	3	2	1	0
11. Another resident/participant has prevented you from accessing resources or services you are entitled to.	4	3	2	1	0
12. Another resident/participant has bossed you around or attempted to control group decision making.	4	3	2	1	0
13. Another resident/participant has made derogatory racial comments to you.	4	3	2	1	0

Figure 4.4. Bullying Questionnaire (Questions 1–10 based on Trompetter, Scholte, & Westerhof [2011]; Questions 11–20 based on Bonifas [2014].) *(Continued)*

From Trompetter, H., Scholte, R., & Westerhof, G. (2011). Resident-to-resident relational aggression and subjective well-being in assisted living facilities. *Aging and Mental Health, 15,* 59–67.
Bonifas, R. P. (January, 2014). Relational aggression in assisted living facilities: Insights into an under-recognized phenomenon. Paper presentation at the 18th Annual Conference of the Society for Social Work Research, San Antonio, Texas.
Appearing in *Bullying Among Older Adults: How to Recognize and Address an Unseen Epidemic,* by Robin P. Bonifas.

14. Another resident/ participant has made derogatory comments to you about your sexual orientation.	4	3	2	1	0
15. Another resident/ participant has made threatening comments to you that made you fearful.	4	3	2	1	0
16. Another resident/ participant has stolen or destroyed your property.	4	3	2	1	0
17. Another resident/ participant has hit, kicked, pinched, pushed, shoved, or bitten you.	4	3	2	1	0
18. Another resident/ participant has intimidated or hurt you with a mobility device, such as a cane, scooter, or electric wheelchair.	4	3	2	1	0
19. Another resident/ participant has been cruel to your pet(s).	4	3	2	1	0
20. Another resident/ participant has intimidated or hurt you with a motor vehicle.	4	3	2	1	0

Figure 4.4. Bullying Questionnaire (Questions 1–10 based on Trompetter, Scholte, & Westerhof [2011]; Questions 11–20 based on Bonifas [2014].)

From Trompetter, H., Scholte, R., & Westerhof, G. (2011). Resident-to-resident relational aggression and subjective well-being in assisted living facilities. *Aging and Mental Health, 15*, 59–67.

Bonifas, R. P. (January, 2014). Relational aggression in assisted living facilities: Insights into an under-recognized phenomenon. Paper presentation at the 18th Annual Conference of the Society for Social Work Research, San Antonio, Texas.

Appearing in *Bullying Among Older Adults: How to Recognize and Address an Unseen Epidemic*, by Robin P. Bonifas.

Bullying Policy Statement

Civil communication is an important part of creating a comfortable living environment at *[insert organization name]*. Our expectation is that everyone who lives here will do his or her part to make others feel at home. In order to accomplish this, frequent use of the following behaviors will be helpful:

- listening
- showing respect
- apologizing
- offering encouragement
- being inclusive
- being agreeable
- welcoming others
- saying "please" and "thank you"

At the same time, living in a communal environment can be difficult and we can sometimes lose patience with our neighbors. If anyone is frustrated or upset in their efforts to create a civil environment, please make an appointment to discuss your concerns in a confidential and safe setting with *[insert name of appointed individual with whom tenants can speak]*.

In helping to create a civil community, please avoid engaging in the following negative behaviors:

- malicious gossiping
- spreading hurtful rumors
- name-calling, mean-spirited teasing, making derogatory remarks
- excluding or attempting to exclude other tenants from activities designed for everyone
- saving seats or tables during meals, activities, or special events
- making offensive gestures or using other negative nonverbal body language toward others, such as mimicking
- making verbal threats to harm others
- stealing
- destroying property
- verbally harassing others
- engaging in any form of physical, verbal, or emotional abuse
- harming or threatening to harm others' pets

If you witness or experience any of the above behaviors, please inform *[insert appointed individual's name]*, who will keep your report confidential and help to resolve the problem.

Because we are serious about creating a safe and comfortable living environment for everyone, engaging in any of the above negative behaviors will result in the following actions: a) 1st offense: verbal and written warnings; b) 2nd offense: verbal and written warnings, discussion with management regarding behavioral improvement strategies; c) 3rd offense: verbal and written warnings, referral to community ombudsman, $25 fine; d) 4th offense: eviction.

Thank you to everyone for consistently striving to create a civil and caring environment at *[insert organization name]*. Let's work together for a positive community!

Figure 4.5. Sample bullying policy statement

CHAPTER 5

Foundational Approaches for People Who Bully

Bullying behavior is often motivated by a need to exercise power and control over others, a need that may be exacerbated among older adults who, as discussed in Chapter 3, can experience overwhelming feelings of loss (in independence, relationships, income, valued roles, social identity, sense of belonging) as well as a lack of empathy or recognition of other's feelings in their transition to assisted living, skilled nursing facilities, and other long-term care settings. Accordingly, the most effective interventions for older adults who bully offer alternative strategies for achieving a sense of personal power and control, help offset feelings of loss, and provide insight into the experiences of others. This chapter outlines strategies to consider, although effective approaches to address bullying will vary from individual to individual and by the type of bullying exhibited.

Consistently Set Limits on Bullying Behaviors

The individual who bullies needs to repeatedly hear that his or her behavior is not acceptable. The person should also clearly and firmly be reminded of his or her boundaries. Consider the following two examples of setting limits, the first in response to a resident wanting the overhead light on in her roommate's space and the second in response to a resident wanting to exclude another resident from a group activity intended to be open to all community members.

Example 1: "Mrs. Jones, I know it's difficult to adjust to a new roommate. However, it violates her rights if you have the overhead light on all night, as it lights her side of the room, too. You're welcome to have a night light for your side of the room instead."

Example 2: "Mrs. Smith, remember that everyone is welcome to play cards during happy hour. Mrs. Cruz, come and sit next to me, and I will help you hold your cards."

Offer an Appropriate Outlet to Vent Frustrations

Sometimes individuals who bully have a difficult time tolerating others who they perceive as different or deviant. These are legitimate feelings. Many older people have not been socialized to welcome diversity to the same extent that people from younger generations have been. As such, it can be helpful to offer a bully who is intolerant an alternative venue to talk about his or her difficulties. For example, meeting one-on-one with a social worker, psychologist, or peer helper to vent frustrations, have those frustrations acknowledged, and then slowly move toward developing strategies to manage the frustrations in ways that do not negatively affect others can help reduce bullying behaviors. Such acknowledgement might look like this:

Resident: I really can't stand individuals from that [cultural group]. I was brought up not to socialize with their kind, and I'm not about to now. Mama always said those people should be avoided at all costs!

Helper: I'm hearing it's really uncomfortable for you to be living with people you were taught not to like. You're feeling put out that there is an expectation to get along with them when doing so has never been your way.

Resident: Right, you really know where I'm coming from.

Helper: I certainly want to respect your point of view. As you know, we need to treat everyone respectfully here, even if they're from walks of life we don't approve of or are uncomfortable with. I'm wondering if it might be helpful for you to talk with me about how unpleasant and difficult it is for you to be living with members of [cultural group], rather than voicing those opinions publically in a way that might be hurtful to others? Might this be a way to compromise on this issue?

After the resident has had an opportunity to express his or her point of view and been received with understanding and without judgment, trust is established. Steps can then be taken to help the resident develop healthier ways of managing negative feelings.

Identify Alternative Methods for People Who Bully to Feel in Control

It is important to help individuals who bully to develop positive methods to feel like they are in control of their environment and situation. Consider the following approach to manage bullying behavior:

> *Example:* A resident was bossing others around by dictating where they could sit and what activities they could participate in. This negative behavior was especially targeted toward individuals who had recently moved into the assisted living community. A staff member began to address the resident's bullying behavior by encouraging her to reflect on how she herself felt when she first moved into the community and the difficulties she had in adjusting to the new setting. The resident reminisced on how that was a rough time for her. The staff member then asked her for help in creating a more welcoming environment for people who had just moved into the apartments. Playing up this individual's potential leadership skills, the staff member encouraged her to devote her energies to organizing a welcome committee. The resident was highly flattered and took on the task with relish. Her bullying behaviors markedly decreased as she became involved in this empowering opportunity.

With some individuals who bully, such efforts can backfire. Careful monitoring is required to ensure that individuals who have engaged in bullying do not use their newfound outlet to further exert controlling behaviors. For example, some individuals might be tempted to create a welcoming committee that purposely excludes others or recruits people into cliques.

Foster the Development of Positive Communication Skills

People are often not familiar with how to speak assertively and are only aware of how to speak aggressively. Individuals who bully may lack skills in expressing wants and needs without hurting others. Helping them to communicate more effectively can reduce bullying behaviors. This can be as simple as teaching the use of "I statements" that emphasize their feelings, as opposed to "you statements" that blame others for problems. Consider this example:

> *Example:* A woman was overheard saying, "Get the hell out of my chair! I told you it was mine for lunch and you could have it at Bingo! Are you deaf or something?!" After being coached by staff, she has learned to instead say "I feel frustrated when I can't sit in my favorite chair. It reminds me of one my husband bought for me long ago. I would like you to let me sit here during lunch; perhaps you can sit here for Bingo."

Similarly, helping individuals who bully to learn the tenets of nonviolent communication can also minimize peer bullying. Nonviolent communication involves expressing one's needs without using negative tactics, such as coercion or threats. It incorporates four elements: observations, feelings, needs, and requests (Rosenberg, 2003). Individuals first state what is bothering them without judgment or evaluation. Then, individuals name the subsequent emotion they are feeling and connect that emotion to an underlying need. Finally, individuals take ownership of meeting their own needs by making a specific request that respects the rights of others. For example, consider the woman in Chapter 4 who loudly repeated *The Lord's Prayer* in her assisted living facility to the chagrin of all of her peers. Rather than screaming at her to shut up, a fellow resident could instead respond by saying, "It's dinner time, and I can hear your voice from across the room. I'm angry about that because I need it to be quieter to enjoy my meal. *The Lord's Prayer* is beautiful, but

I wonder if you'd be willing to repeat it quietly to yourself instead." Readers are encouraged to learn more about nonviolent communication strategies through the Center for Nonviolent Communication at http://www.cnvc.org.

Help People Who Bully Expand Their Social Network

Not surprising, individuals who bully have few friends, which can complicate matters. A bully may rationalize his or her behavior by thinking, "Why bother being respectful when no one likes me anyway?" Helping bullies connect with others in positive ways can help bolster self-esteem and provide motivation for behavioral change. Introductions centered on shared interests or experiences are a good way to begin. Introducing bullies to online social networking opportunities can also be helpful to beginning forming a sense of positive connection with others.

Foster the Development of Empathy

Individuals who bully often lack empathy. Fortunately, research suggests that empathy can be learned (Beddoe & Murphy, 2004; Siegel, 2007). Modeling is one method for fostering empathy and involves sharing reflections with a bully on how a target may have felt related to a bullying incident and then inviting the bully to elaborate on those feelings. For example, a senior care provider might say, "I noticed Brenda looked very sad when you said her new hairdo looked like a demented bird's nest in front of the quilters' group. What other feelings do you think Brenda may have felt when you said what you said to her?" Having the target tell the bully directly how he or she felt, with a trusted individual present to provide support and safety for both individuals, can also be especially powerful. However, it is important to recognize that not all targets will welcome such a challenging encounter.

Empathy Training

Empathy has been suggested as one of the best antidotes to relational aggression and other bullying behaviors (Richardson, Hommock, Smith, Gardner, & Manuel, 1994). Defined as the capacity to understand and share in another's emotional experience (Jolliffe & Farrington, 2004), empathy is linked to compassionate behaviors and is recognized as a skill that can be learned (Riess, Kelley, Bailey, Dunn, & Phillips, 2012). Indeed, research has identified mirror neurons that mediate empathy in the brain whereby "when we see another person's actions (e.g., laughing or crying), our bodies respond as if we feel a degree of that action, too" (Gerdes & Segal, 2009, p. 117). Empathy training is one approach for further conditioning this innate mirroring and has been effective in increasing positive interactions and reducing negative interactions among various groups, including nurses (Cunico, Sartori, Marognolli, & Meneghini, 2012), resident physicians (Riess et al., 2012), and schoolchildren (Sahin, 2012). As such, this approach holds promise for yielding similar results among older adults.

Grounded in neuroscience, training incorporates the cognitive and affective components of empathy (Decety & Moriguchi, 2007):

- affective sharing or reflecting on another's observable experience

- self-awareness or purposefully recognizing one's own emotional experience

- mental flexibility or imagining the world from another's perspective

- emotional regulation or moderating emotions stemming from mirroring another's experience

Empathy training is often combined with mindfulness practice to bolster learners' ability to attend to their emotional and physical states in the here and now (Gerdes & Segal, 2009; Riess et al, 2012). Mindfulness practice, or intentionally being present in the moment without judgment (Kabat-Zinn, 1994), has been deemed a beneficial approach in fostering psychosocial well-being among a wide range of older adults (McBee, 2008). Furthermore, mindfulness-based activities are primarily experiential and can be delivered by trained paraprofessional staff with professional guidance. Chapter 8 presents a detailed empathy training program.

Table 5.1 summarizes intervention options available to care providers based on the type of bullying behaviors exhibited.

Table 5.1. Bullying behaviors and associated interventions.

Bullying behavior or associated context	Suggested intervention
Verbal bullying and relational aggression, such as excluding, gossiping, name-calling, mimicking, and derogatory remarks	Set limits.
Bullying behavior associated with difficulty tolerating differences, such as derogatory racial statements or comments about sexual orientation, socioeconomic status, or religious views	Offer an appropriate outlet to vent frustrations.
Domineering, bossing, and controlling others, blocking access to services or commodities available to all members of the community	Provide healthy alternatives to feel in control.
Bullying others when angry, frustrated, or upset in response to a behavior a person finds annoying	Promote positive communication skills.
Bully has few friends with limited motivation for positive interaction because he or she feels unliked anyway	Expand social network.
Bully has limited insight into how his or her behaviors impact others and sees no reason to change behavior	Provide empathy training.
Bullying behaviors do not respond to intervention and pose a severe risk of harm to other residents/ participants or significantly violates others' civil rights	Offer mediation. Then consider discharging or evicting the bully.

Ethical Challenges that Can Arise in Bullying Situations among Older Adults

As with any human phenomenon, there are ethical issues associated with striving to manage bullying behaviors among older adults. This section addresses the following five ethical challenges:

- organizational inaction

- unequal or biased resident treatment

- protecting residents' rights

- working with extraordinarily difficult residents

- addressing bullying in the context of mental health conditions

Because ethical dilemmas, by definition, have no single correct resolution, this section provides readers with contexts for how to think about difficult issues, not specific answers to ethical problems.

Organizational Inaction

Some senior care organizations are reluctant to take a proactive stance against bullying. For example, Doris Lor, a 76-year-old resident of a retirement community, describes ongoing episodes of being excluded by other residents from using community resources or attending events (Creno, 2010): "There is a clique here that is meaner than mean . . . The first time I went to the recreation center, a man yelled at me, 'This is a private club. You aren't welcome here.'" In spite of repeated episodes of bullying, Ms. Lor reports she did not receive any support from community administration and even "receive[d] a letter of reprimand from the [Homeowners Association] . . . after she tried to confront the residents she says [were excluding] her from community programs . . . Despite repeated complaints and letters to the director of her homeowners association, she can't get a seat at a card table, gets the cold shoulder at the women's club, and has been chased away from seats at the community pool."

At times, the perception that *it's just the way people are* or *there's nothing that can be done* influences organizational inaction. At other times, organizational passivity is related to a belief that bullying is merely a social irritant and does not cause any lasting harm. However, nothing is further from the truth. Organizational personnel may also perceive that managing bullying behaviors is the residents' responsibility, not that of the organization, and, therefore, refrain from taking action in a misguided attempt to promote resident independence. This is akin to expecting students on the playground to be in charge of bullying prevention without any support from teachers and administrators. As discussed in Chapter 4, a three-tiered approach that includes the bully, the target of bullying, and the organization is necessary to address bullying. Keep in mind that living in an environment where bullying is allowed to occur creates a culture of fear, disrespect, and insecurity and can actually lead to increased bullying. Such environments also reduce resident satisfaction (Bonifas & Frankel, 2012).

Unequal or Biased Resident Treatment

Organizational personnel are human and, naturally, like some residents better than others. There is nothing wrong with this, of course, unless it contributes to disparate treatment of residents. In the case of bullying, individuals who bully may not exhibit negative behaviors in the presence of people in authority. Therefore, administrators may be surprised to learn that seemingly nice individuals engage in bullying behaviors and may not take complaints about such behavior seriously. On the other hand, with residents who are outwardly unpleasant toward most people, administrative staff may be overly harsh in attempts to curtail bullying behaviors. The same is true for the targets of bullying. Those who are well liked may get a more rapid and effective response than those who are among the staff's least favorites.

To minimize the risk of treating residents unequally, staff must avoid making decisions in isolation about how to address bullying. Rather, they should investigate what happened by interviewing all of those involved, including the bully, target, and witnesses; discuss the situation with colleagues; and determine a course of action as a team.

Protecting Residents' Rights

People have a right to live in an environment that promotes the highest quality of life possible, which includes an environment free from bullying. However, individuals also have the right to their own opinions and may voice those opinions, as long as in doing so they don't verbally attack their peers' personal attributes, qualities, or beliefs. Similarly, people have a right to be who they are, feel what they feel, and have a bad day now and again.

For example, Edward, a resident in assisted living who holds strong negative beliefs about homosexuality, often makes his opinions known in public areas of the facility and usually in response to media coverage of gay and lesbian issues. He makes comments such as "I don't hold with same-sex relations" or "I don't approve of homosexuality," but does not direct those comments to anyone in particular. Such statements are considered politically incorrect and are certainly in poor taste, but they cannot be considered bullying. There are no underlying issues of power involved, nor is there a specific target. Yet, gay and lesbian residents who hear his comments likely feel uncomfortable and unwelcome in the environment, which is not conducive to promoting quality of life and creating a caring community for all.

So how should organizational personnel handle the conflicting needs of Edward and gay and lesbian residents? The first step is to recognize that Edward is entitled to his own views about homosexuality. The goal of intervention is not to change his opinions or criticize his beliefs, but to help him express his beliefs in a way that does not infringe on the well-being of others. In this case, it would be important to encourage Edward to set limits on where he shares such opinions; that is, not in community areas of the building, but perhaps as part of a forum on "hot" topics or social issues where attendance is by choice.

It is not realistic to expect everyone to be on her or his best behavior 100% of the time. Everyone has an off day now and again. In addition, there is variability in people's social relationship patterns. Some individuals are naturally nice and friendly, while others are more reserved or even surly. In managing bullying behaviors, organizational personnel need to allow people to be who they are and recognize that someone who is having an off day or is perhaps always gruff toward others is not necessarily a bully.

Working with Extraordinarily Difficult Residents

There may be circumstances in which an individual who bullies is simply too difficult to manage. Staff members may try multiple interventions and hold repeated resident and family meetings without subsequent behavioral change. Alternatively, the resident may refuse all recommended interventions. In these highly difficult situations, the individual who bullies may have a substance abuse history, a serious mental illness, or experienced severe trauma in the past. He or she may not be suited for living in senior housing or participating in senior center environments. In these extreme cases, it is prudent to consider an alternative environment in which the bully's needs can be met. Because the individual is likely to refuse to relocate voluntarily, documentation of ongoing problems, intervention efforts, and the impact of bullying behavior on facility residents is critical. Administrative personnel may wish to consult with outside experts to determine the best course of action, such as ombudspersons, corporate leaders, and provider advocacy organizations.

Bullying in the Context of Mental Health Conditions

Aggressive and other challenging behaviors stemming from mental health conditions are not usually considered bullying because such symptoms are not exclusively motivated by needs for power and control. In fact, because assisted living residents report being fearful of peers' disruptive psychiatric symptoms, individuals with mental health conditions are likely to be the *targets* of bullying. Indeed, individuals with mental illness already face considerable stigma. Care providers can minimize magnifying these residents' feelings of shame by avoiding negative profiling or labeling them as inherently dangerous. Rather, it is prudent to use a universal precautions approach and to keep in mind the potential for any resident to be involved in bullying, regardless of mental health status. This is especially advisable given that psychiatric conditions may not be disclosed, may be undiagnosed, or may develop after a resident moves in. That said, it is important to act quickly if any of the warning signs listed at the end of Chapter 3 are present. Chapters 4 and 8 describe potential courses of action.

In the context of mental health disorders, behavior that resembles bullying is typically linked to decreased impulse control or distorted perceptions that lead to a sense of feeling threatened. As described by Algase and colleagues (1996) in relation to people with dementia, such "bullies" may have difficulty negotiating or communicating their needs. In contrast to traditional bullying, rather than trying to usurp others' power, these individuals may be trying to gain a feeling of control over a distressing situation or chaotic environment in the only way they know how. Even so, it is important to recognize that mental health conditions can complicate bullying situations and heighten the complexity of determining interventions. For example, in the nursing home tragedy mentioned in Chapter 1, Ms. Lindquist's mental health status may have contributed to the bullying behavior that led to Ms. Barrow's murder. In this case, Ms. Lindquist's delusional beliefs about her roommate's intention to monopolize the shared room space caused her to feel threatened, and she acted aggressively in a misguided effort to protect herself. The key issue here is that the delusional beliefs represent the primary problem and should be the target for intervention, rather than simply the aggressive behavior alone. With mental health disorders, the underlying condition must be addressed; with actual bullying, the individual's need for power must be addressed and limits must be set on acceptable ways to achieve a sense of control. It is essential to note that the distinction between symptoms of mental illness and bullying would hardly be meaningful to Ms. Barrow

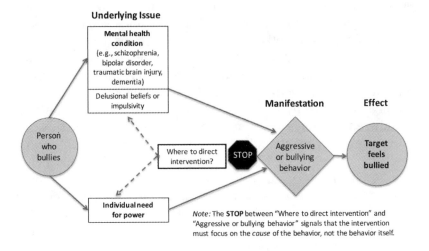

Figure 5.1. Relationships among factors associated with bullying behaviors, interventions, and outcomes.

or her family. Regardless of the motivation behind the behavior, it feels like bullying to be on the receiving end of such negativity, and even more so considering the horrific outcome in this specific case. Figure 5.1 summarizes the distinctions between behaviors associated with mental illness and bullying and where interventions should be directed in both cases (i.e., the underlying cause of the behavior rather than the behavior itself).

Symptoms associated with schizophrenia, bipolar disorder, traumatic brain injury, and dementia can make individuals prone to exhibiting bullying or bullying-like behaviors or to being targeted by others. For instance, schizophrenia contributes to disordered thinking, a distorted sense of reality, hallucinations, delusions, a limited range of emotional expression, and poor social skills. With bipolar disorder, someone in the manic phase commonly experiences poor judgment, difficulty managing one's temper, lack of self-control, excessive activity, and grandiose beliefs about oneself. Traumatic brain injury leads to memory and concentration difficulties, mood changes and swings, agitation, aggressiveness, and impulsivity. Similarly, dementia causes cognitive impairments that can contribute to negative behaviors, including aggression and intrusiveness. Dementia-related behaviors in particular, including wandering into others' rooms or rummaging through others' personal items, can trigger reciprocal bullying.

Older adults with mental health conditions sometimes believe that they are being bullied when in fact bullying is not occurring. Strong emotional reactions to peers' minor social faux pas may also be exhibited. For example, an older adult with bipolar disorder had this response to being accidently bumped in the elevator by a male peer whom she did not like:

> "I have to kick the fire alarm button if he's going up the elevator because he will altercate me . . . I have to try and avoid being harangued or disabled. I'm multiply disabled . . . if he hits me, and I fall, I'll break a bone. That's it; I'll be dead. Within a year, I'll be dead" (Bonifas, 2011).

Summary

This chapter discussed basic interventions that can help minimize bullying behaviors among older adults and reviewed how to identify which intervention might be most appropriate in a given situation. Interventions include setting limits, providing appropriate outlets to vent feelings of frustration, identifying alternative healthy strategies for bullies to feel in control, and helping individuals who bully to develop positive communication skills, expand their social networks, and be empathetic toward others. Ethical challenges that can arise as part of anti-bullying interventions were also discussed. Chapter 6 describes foundational approaches to help those older adults who are the targets of peer bullying.

Foundational Approaches for People Who Are Bullied

Empowering Targets to Thwart Bullying

The interventions discussed in this chapter are intended for the targets of bullying who have sufficient cognitive abilities to learn new skills to minimize others' ability to dominate them. Comfort levels in learning and practicing such skills will vary across individuals. Those who are generally passive by nature will have more difficulty than those who are normally assertive but who are stymied by the new experience of being bullied. Regardless, it is often best to start with the following small behavioral changes and then gradually increase residents' self-advocacy skills:

Step 1: Gain comfort and confidence in reporting bullying incidents to authority figures. This can begin by staff regularly checking in with residents to assess whether bullying has occurred. If it has, help the target report an incident in writing or verbally. Verbal reports may be more effective if the target first practices reporting with a trusted individual before making the report to administrative personnel.

Step 2: Exert more control in preventing bullying incidents by positioning oneself out of harm's way. Help individuals select seating that offers an escape from a bully. For example, sitting near exits or near staff members or volunteers can minimize instances of bullying.

Step 3: Verbally respond to bullies in increasingly sophisticated ways that minimize their power over the individual. Help a target to plan simple things to say to thwart a bully's power, such as, "The activity coordinator said seats shouldn't be saved, so I am going to sit here. You might talk with the activity coordinator if you're unhappy about that." Or "I know we're working to develop a caring community, and calling me a fat pig isn't in keeping with that. See you later." As with reporting bullying incidents, it is helpful if the target first practices such responses with a trusted individual.

Note that simply telling individuals about these strategies or describing things to say to bullies is insufficient in teaching them to develop self-advocacy skills. It is essential to practice such skills by role-playing so that they actually learn how to use them. Only through practice and experience do skills develop. Role-playing is a learning technique in which the senior care provider plays the part of the bully and the resident practices empowering responses. Ongoing feedback from the care provider will enhance an older adult's feelings of mastery and confidence in responding to a bully.

Reporting Incidents

Some individuals are reluctant to report bullying incidents for fear of reprisal or drawing attention. Indeed, they do not even feel powerful enough to make their needs known. Therefore, helping them to become comfortable with reporting incidents to authority figures, such as administrative personnel or police officers, is an important initial goal. It is also essential that that person in authority takes the reporting and concerns seriously and follows up to minimize feelings of being targeted.

As noted in Chapter 4, policies and procedures for reporting are helpful. Recognize that some residents may wish to make face-to-face reports and others may be more comfortable making written reports. It is vital to develop reporting forms that cue objective statements regarding the facts of what happened. For example, it is much more useful to have a report that reads "Mabel Jones told me after lunch on Friday that I couldn't play Bingo with the group because it's only for smart people and no dummies are allowed," rather than "Mabel Jones was mean to me after lunch." Chapter 7 provides an example written report form that readers will find useful.

Even with encouragement from administrative staff, some residents still feel reluctant to report problems. A useful strategy is to appeal to their sense of concern for others by saying something like, "I know it's no fun to voice complaints or concerns about others, but if Mr. Thomas is behaving that way toward you, it's likely that he's treating others poorly as well. Your willingness to make this problem known might help everyone feel more comfortable in getting help."

When practicing with a resident, first have him or her describe a hypothetical incident of bullying. Once the person has gained a level of comfort with that, then move on to reporting a real incident that happened in the past. Both of these practice situations are devoid of fear of retaliation. After an actual bullying incident occurs, the target could then practice making his or her report with a care provider before actually reporting it to someone in a position of authority.

Positioning Oneself Out of Harm's Way

Once an individual is able to confidently report problems, the next step is to help him or her exert more positive control in preventing bullying incidents. One way to accomplish this is to teach the person to position him- or herself out of harm's way, not by self-isolation, avoiding activities of interest, or taking long circuitous routes around problem individuals, but by attending group events as usual and sitting near activity leaders or protective peers. For example, during bingo, the individual might sit near the person calling the numbers, or during a musical event, he or she might choose a seat near the entertainer. These approaches are helpful because bullying individuals are less likely to cause problems when people outside the resident community are watching. Another strategy is to sit near a peer who won't tolerate bullying and can thus act as an advocate. This can also inspire the target to feel more confident in asking a bully to stop his or her negative behavior. Peers who have mastered the bystander intervention strategies described in Chapter 7 are excellent helpers in this role.

In addition, teach the target to identify seats that provide easy opportunities to move away from a bully. Rather than getting cornered sitting in a back table against the wall, encourage the person to sit near entryways or by a communication device that quickly allows him or her to call for help.

Making Verbal Responses to Thwart a Bully's Power

Individuals who are the target of bullying must develop communication skills that prevent the bully from achieving power over them. This is typically accomplished through brief verbal responses that deflate the bully's efforts by drawing attention to his or her shortcomings without engaging in retaliatory bullying. For example, when a bully says "Hey, fatso! Was that an Earth tremor I felt earlier, or did you walk by?" the target might say "Well, if you don't know what an earthquake feels like, maybe you should research the topic a bit further," and then simply walk away. Similarly, when a bully comments negatively on a target's hairdo, he or she might say, "Well, that may be true, but members of polite society don't say things like that."

Referring to organizational policies and procedures or authority figures when being bullied can also help the target to retain power. For example, when a bully or group of bullies tries to claim all of the seating around the fireplace or the best seats for religious services, the target can say, "Remember, we have a no-saving seats policy here. I'm sure you wouldn't forget something like that." Or "The resident services manager stated seats were first come, first serve. If you're unhappy that I won't move from this seat, I suggest you speak with her about your concern." Statements that reference a third party also help targets draw attention away from themselves and can enhance comfort with self-advocacy.

Learning to set limits with peers who make unreasonable demands is another helpful strategy. For example, when a peer continually hounds someone for money, the targeted individual might say something like, "I would like to help you, but you haven't paid me back from the last loan I gave you. After you've paid me back, I'll feel more comfortable loaning to you again in the future." If the person continues to exert pressure, the target can then say "I won't discuss this further until you're able to pay me back for the last time; those are the rules."

Confronting the individual who bullies about his or her behavior is another effective approach to prevent them from gaining power. The target can describe the impact of the bullying behavior in an assertive manner, such as by saying "When you tell me that I'm not allowed to join in the card game because my hands shake too much, I feel hurt and excluded. I think you need to make allowances for the limitations of others so that more people can join the game." It is important to note that some individuals have difficulty differentiating assertive behavior from aggressive behavior. If this distinction is not clear, people who are the targets of bullying may likely bully others in return. Teaching a target of bullying to make "I" statements and use nonviolent communication approaches, as described in Chapter 7, are also useful strategies in practicing assertiveness and emphasizing how being assertive is different from being aggressive.

When role-playing with a resident, ask the person to reconstruct aggressive, confrontational statements, such as "You make me so mad" or "You are such an insensitive person," into assertive statements: "When you raise your voice at the table during mealtime, I have difficulty enjoying my meal." Or "When you imitate the way I talk, I feel angry and embarrassed."

It is important to remember that individuals who are targeted by bullies often have low self-esteem. Therefore, helping them to foster their self-worth and dignity is essential. Make special efforts to notice and comment on an individual's strengths and showcase those strengths to others, as appropriate. Involve them in activities and projects that provide a sense of accomplishment. Ensure that they are able to get to the barber or beauty shop to have their nails done or beard trimmed—all of those little things that help people to feel good about themselves.

Support Groups

Usually if bullying is occurring in senior housing settings or senior centers, more than one individual is targeted. Bringing these individuals together as a formal group to both support one another and teach new skills to handle bullies is extremely beneficial. The following outlines an 8-week plan to develop such a support group:

Session 1: Discuss the definition of bullying. Encourage participants to share how it feels to be disempowered and to support one another in sharing their experiences.

Session 2: Discuss the different types of bullying. Encourage participants to share which types of bullying they have experienced and to support one another in sharing their experiences.

Session 3: Discuss the characteristics of bullies and the targets of bullying. Review anti-bullying and self-advocacy skills that participants can be taught. Encourage participants to share anti-bullying skills that they would like to learn and to support one another in sharing their experiences.

Session 4: Discuss strategies to counteract bullying. Practice skills via role-play.

Session 5: Continue to discuss strategies to counteract bullying. Practice skills via role-play.

Session 6: Continue to discuss strategies to counteract bullying. Practice skills via role-play.

Session 7: Discuss progress in responding to bullies. Mutually support one another's efforts.

Session 8: Closing celebration. Encourage participants to discuss plans for continued self-empowerment.

Interventions for People Who Misperceive Being the Targets of Bullying

Some people think they are being bullied, when in fact they are not. This can happen with individuals who are emotionally sensitive, who have limited understanding of others' psychiatric conditions, or who are struggling with a mental health condition. For these individuals, additional approaches can be beneficial.

First, psychoeducation can help those who are upset by outward symptoms of mental health disorders, such as when a peer carries on loud conversations with unseen stimuli. Psychoeducation provides information that helps the person better understand what is going on, which reduces fear and anxiety. Of course, such information needs to be provided in a manner that protects the confidentiality of the individual exhibiting the symptoms. For example, it would not be appropriate to say, "Mr. Jameson has schizophrenia and has hallucinations whereby he thinks God is giving him advice. He takes medications to control his more challenging symptoms and won't harm anyone." Such an explanation violates HIPAA privacy regulations (Health Insurance Portability and Accountability Act of 1996). A more appropriate approach would be to share through a brief educational workshop general information about schizophrenia and hallucinations without indicating that any specific individual living in the community has the condition or symptoms. For example, workshops on "Understanding Auditory Hallucinations" or "Coping with Dementia" would be appropriate. Then, when incidents do occur, quietly and privately remind those individuals who voice concerns about the workshops. For example: "That does sound pretty disruptive, but remember what we learned in the workshop last week? People who wander are usually having difficulty locating the restroom and don't realize they're violating your privacy. How did the person who led the workshop suggest you handle this situation?"

Senior care organization personnel who do not have the expertise to provide such workshops might consider contracting with a mental health professional, such as a psychologist, social worker, or nurse. Alternatively, the *Hearing Voices That Are Distressing* curriculum offers an excellent program for developing sensitivity toward individuals who experience auditory hallucinations. Interested readers can find out more through the National Empowerment Center, Inc. (http://www.power2u.org/mm5/merchant.mvc).

For those who are highly emotionally sensitive, using a combination of validation, setting limits, and requesting help is useful. It is important to acknowledge the individual's distress so that he or she feels heard rather than ignored. At the same time, however, senior care providers will want to discourage emotionally sensitive reactions by not rewarding the individual with extra personal attention and thereby encouraging his or her reactions. Validation involves first commenting on the individual's emotional state: "Ms. Valdez, I can tell you're really upset about what happened in the elevator. It sounds like that was a difficult experience for you. It's no fun to be bumped into." Next, point out an alternative explanation for what happened: "I have the sense that Mr. Jorge didn't mean to hurt you and that bumping you was not intentional." Follow this with a request for help in managing the situation: "Because you have not been physically harmed, I wonder if you might help me out by considering this an accident and forgiving Mr. Jorge for his mistake?" Acknowledging the situation and then turning it back to the individual in this manner helps minimize the potential for emotionally needy people to monopolize staff time with repetitive erroneous complaints.

This approach is also useful in working with individuals whose perception of being bullied stems from underlying mental health conditions. In conjunction, it is also necessary to ensure that the disorder is treated appropriately, perhaps with a referral to the individual's physician or a contracted mental health provider.

People with Dementia Who Are Bullied

In discussing interventions to address individuals who are bullied, it is important to acknowledge that people with dementia who are bullied require different interventions from those who do not have dementia. Dementia impairs cognition such that individuals in the middle stages of the disease progression are not able to learn new skills due to severely limited short-term memory. Thus, interventions cannot be based on *teaching* these individuals how to deal with bullies. Rather, staff members must monitor individuals with dementia and redirect them from harm's way. Environmental modifications can, of course, also help. Examples include using visual barriers to prevent wanderers from entering into others' rooms or creating circular pathways to support wandering in areas that are not inappropriate. Readers can refer to the Alzheimer's Association website for resources on protecting individuals with dementia (https://www.alz.org).

When Residents Target Staff

Employees of senior housing and senior care organizations are also troubled by residents' bullying behaviors and often report feeling overwhelmed by trying to manage negative interactions. This frustration is associated with both resident-to-resident bullying and residents who bully staff members. In one example, an assisted living resident repeatedly told a worker that she could not speak English properly and he would see to it that she was fired (Bonifas & Frankel, 2012). In another example, an older assisted living resident repeatedly harassed a young social worker, calling her incompetent and highlighting her inexperience when she tried to enforce facility rules (Bonifas & Frankel, 2012). Some staff members are particularly vulnerable to bullying from the residents in their care. These include younger workers who are still developing experience and confidence as well as workers who, relative to the organization's clientele, are a part of minority groups. Staff members often fear reporting bullying incidents to supervisors due to perceptions that they may put their job at risk, and they often are uncomfortable setting limits for residents or participants who bully them because they fear violating clients' rights. As such, training for staff on how to manage bullying situations is as necessary as training residents and participants themselves. The following are important elements of an introductory staff anti-bullying training. Chapter 9 provides a detailed staff intervention program that offers more advanced content.

1. Overview of bullying among older adults

2. Review of organizational policies and procedures for addressing bullying and relational aggression between residents and toward staff

3. Bystander intervention skills (Alcon, Barnes, & Frankel [2014])

4. Respect for clients' rights: limit-setting, nonviolent communication, strategies to retain power

5. How and when to make a report

6. Assurances of an overall caring community approach that protects residents and staff

Administrative support is vital in enabling staff to effectively respond to residents or participants who bully. Staff reports of bullying must be be met with consideration and a quick response. Individuals who bully may be resentful of staff members who set limits on their behavior and may respond with reciprocal bullying or may retaliate by complaining about the staff member to management, potentially resulting in a situation whereby management aligns with the resident and the staff member gets in trouble for trying to counteract bullying behaviors. This situation only proves to perpetuate the cycle. Therefore, it is imperative that management, staff, and residents collaborate in addressing bullying situations, whether peer bullying or bullying of staff.

Summary

This chapter discussed several promising interventions to empower individuals who are targeted by bullies. General approaches include anti-bullying support groups and strategies to help targets in developing assertiveness and communication skills to prevent a bully from achieving power over them as well as to become comfortable with reporting incidents to authority figures. The chapter also described staff anti-bullying training for cases in which a resident bullies a staff member. Chapter 7 begins the section on detailed interventions to address bullying among older adults, and features an assessment strategy as well as three step-by-step interventions: "upstander" training, resident recognition programs, and pro-social activities.

PART III

Creating Caring Communities

Bullying Assessment Strategies and Interventions

~~~~~~

Eleanor Feldman Barbera

This chapter offers a comprehensive approach to preventing bullying among older adults in long-term care settings such as assisted living facilities and nursing homes. The section "Assessing the Situation" examines strategies to assess, report, and track bullying within an organization, and the section "Bullying Interventions" discusses three interconnected prevention interventions to minimize negative interactions. The first-level intervention trains staff and residents to identify bullying and to be "upstanders" rather than bystanders when bullying behavior is observed. The second-level intervention uses recognition programs to reward positive interactions among residents. Lastly, the third-level intervention centers on involving long-term care community members in positive, pro-social activities to create a more empathic environment where older adults have less time for engaging in negative behaviors. Of the three, upstander training is the most crucial prevention strategy for the community.

Assessing the Situation: Conduct an Initial Assessment

A review of assisted living communities by Margaret Wylde, Ph.D., and the American Seniors Housing Association (Unlocking the Mystery of Very Satisfied Independent Living Customers: Make

Them "Feel at Home," 2014) found that bullying occurred in every community included in the study. Given this finding, bullying is likely present in your senior care organization as well. An assessment of the existence and extent of bullying within your community will help in targeting interventions to the exact nature of the relationship difficulties that exist among residents and participants.

Tool #1: Social Interaction Survey

The first part of the assessment process is gathering information from community residents using the Social Interaction Survey (see the Appendix). The survey asks questions about the types of bullying that are occurring, the locations, and the individuals involved, along with other pertinent information. Originally used with children in schools settings, the survey is adapted from the work of Rodney Pruitt, M.A., a consultant for school districts in west Texas in safety and drug-use prevention efforts. The assessment tool can be used as is or further adapted to the specifics of your organization. For example, if you suspect there may be a specific area in which bullies are targeting others, a question can be added about feelings of safety in that particular location. If your community has an active social media presence, a question might be included regarding bullying using those forums. This questionnaire is more comprehensive than the one presented in Chapter 4 (see Figure 4.4) in that it includes questions about where and when bullying behaviors occur, elicits residents' input on the bullying experiences of others as well as their own, and asks residents how they responded to negative behaviors. It is a good second-level assessment for organizations that are ready for more advanced understanding of the bullying behaviors occurring within their community.

It is important to consider readability when using written surveys with older adults, many of whom have difficulty reading small type and relatively ornate fonts. To increase the likelihood that your community members will be able to complete the questionnaire independently, use the following recommendations from the American Foundation for the Blind to enhance readability:

- *Print type size:* Use an 18-point type size; a 16-point type size is the minimum.

- *Font type and style:* Use standard Roman or sans serif fonts, such as Arial and Helvetica. Use bold type and avoid italics.

- *Leading (space between lines of text):* Rather than single-spacing the document, use 1.5 spaces between lines.

(For a copy of the survey following these print guidelines, contact the author of this chapter at drel@mybetternursinghome.com.)

Administering the Social Interaction Survey

Ideally, community residents and staff will complete the survey independently. If residents are unable to complete the surveys on their own, staff members can assist, using as private a location as possible to gather accurate information. Keep in mind that some-one who is being bullied may feel too intimidated by the presence of a bully to truthfully answer the question aloud, such as in the case of a resident being surveyed in the presence of a bullying roommate. In addition, residents may be uncomfortable voicing concerns to staff members for fear of being labeled a complainer or "tattletale." To avoid these concerns, consider bringing in peo-ple from outside of the community, such as local university stu-dents of nursing, social work, or psychology, to administer the survey as your budget allows.

To ensure that most questionnaires are returned, distribute and collect them as part of a group meeting, perhaps one that dis-cusses neighborly behavior or the issue of bullying. The following steps detail how to present the survey in a group meeting format prior to distribution to residents:

1. Hold a meeting with staff members to review and discuss the questionnaire and answer any questions and concerns they might have regarding its use. This will allow for a smoother distribution to the residents.

2. Next, hold a meeting with both staff and residents to explain the purpose of the questionnaire. Make the following points:

   - The intent of the survey is to ensure that the community is a safe and friendly place for all residents.

   - The survey will be used to identify any problem areas in order to make improvements in community life.

   - The survey will collect information about social interac-tions between residents and *not* between staff members and residents.

- The information that residents share will not be shared with other residents without their permission, and any identified problems will be handled individually and confidentially (unless someone is in physical danger).

Once the questionnaires have been completed, use the following guidelines for what to do with the survey results:

- Staff members should assess areas of the community noted to be prone to bullying and take actions to reduce its likelihood. For example, if bullying is occurring in the dining room, seating may need to be altered. If bullying is taking place during activities, recreation staff may need specific strategies to deter negative interactions in those situations.

- In order to maintain confidentiality, use discretion in identifying bullies. Consider the survey results a starting point for closer observation of how identified residents interact with others as well as for gentle, individual discussions with them.

- For those noted to be targets of bullying, speak with them privately about their experiences and offer counseling, support, and coping strategies. For example, someone who is targeted during activity groups might be encouraged to sit closer to the facilitator.

- For those noted to be bullies, speak with them privately to address others' perceptions of their actions. Avoid assuming that they are intentionally engaging in bullying behaviors.

- Many bullies do not know they are perceived as such and may need compassionate counseling as well as training in social skills to develop alternative methods of relating to others. Local mental health providers can provide information about social skills training, if necessary.

Tool #2: Bullying Incident Report Form

Along with assessing the nature of and extent to which bullying is occurring in your organization, it is also helpful to track how often such behaviors occur. A Bullying Incident Report Form can be used to log incidents of bullying (see the Appendix).

Tool #3: Ongoing Bullying Report Form

Just as many senior care organizations have to complete forms if falls occur, a form can be used to track recurring incidents of bullying behaviors as well as identify patterns and repeat offenders, as in the example that follows. A completed report form (using details from individual incident reports) might include the information shown in Figure 7.1, which is based on a school bullying assessment form developed by Rodney Pruitt.

Date	Aggressor	Target	Location	Time	Behavior
12/20/16	Ms. Fox	Ms. Patel	Dining room	5:10pm	Taunting
12/20/16	Ms. Cohen	Mr. Smith	Lounge	2:45pm	Teasing, criticizing
12/21/16	Ms. Jones	Ms. Lupo	E wing hall	8:20am	Gossiping
12/21/16	Ms. Johnson	Ms. Lupo	E wing hall	8:20am	Gossiping
12/21/16	Ms. Fox	Ms. Patel	Dining room	5:20pm	Taunting
12/22/16	Ms. Jones	Mr. Smith	Dining room	12:10pm	Yelling, threatening
12/22/16	Ms. Diaz	Mr. Smith	Dining room	12:10pm	Yelling, threatening
12/22/16	Ms. Johnson	Mr. Smith	Dining room	12:10pm	Hitting
12/23/16	Ms. Fox	Ms. Patel	Dining room	5:15pm	Taunting, threatening
12/24/16	Ms. Jones	Ms. Day	Lounge	2:40pm	Gossiping, threatening
12/24/16	Ms. Diaz	Ms. Day	Lounge	2:40pm	Gossiping, threatening
12/24/16	Mr. Connell	Ms. Jones	Lounge	2:45pm	Yelling, threatening
12/24/16	Mr. Connell	Ms. Diaz	Lounge	2:45pm	Yelling, threatening
12/24/16	Ms. Fox	Ms. Patel	Dining room	5:10pm	Threatening, pushing

Figure 7.1. Sample completed Ongoing Bullying Report Form.

Examination of the tracking form by the care team can illuminate patterns. Look for the following:

- **Residents observed to bully on more than one occasion.** In the sample tracking form, a group of bullies appears to exist consisting of Ms. Jones, Ms. Diaz, and sometimes Ms. Johnson. They are bullying several residents in more than one location.

- **Residents who appear to be bullying the bulliers.** On 12/24, Mr. Connell bullied Ms. Jones and Ms. Diaz; perhaps he was standing up for Ms. Day. Note that 5 minutes of bullying had occurred without staff intervention, so he may have felt compelled to act because no staff had intervened. Mr. Connell does not appear to be bullying other residents.

- **Patterns of bullying between two residents.** Ms. Fox has been bullying Ms. Patel on an ongoing and intensifying basis.

- **Residents who are being bullied by more than one individual or group of people.** Mr. Smith has been targeted by more than one bully or bullying group.

- **The location of the bullying.** A great deal of bullying is occurring in the dining room during mealtimes.

- **The timing of the bullying and outside events that might be triggering distress among the residents.** The incidents in the sample tracking form are occurring just prior to Christmas, so perhaps those involved are particularly troubled regarding family issues or are experiencing feelings of loss that are common around the holidays. Other triggers could be the departure of a favorite staff member or peer, or world events that raise anxiety.

Once staff have assessed the information in the tracking form, it can be used to develop interventions, such as the following:

- Discuss with Ms. Jones, Ms. Diaz, and Ms. Johnson their behaviors.

- Change seating or increase staff presence in the dining room.

- Train staff to identify and intervene in bullying situations so that other residents do not feel compelled to get involved.

- Observe and counsel Mr. Smith to address his being bullied by peers.

- Discuss interactions individually with Ms. Fox and Ms. Patel.

- Hold a community workshop to discuss the challenges of the holidays and ways to handle feelings of grief and loss.

Bullying Interventions

Once an assessment of bullying has been completed within the community and it is determined that interventions are necessary, consider implementing the following three-pronged approach.

First-Level Intervention: How to Become an "Upstander"

Whereas bystanders watch silently while others are bullied, upstanders intervene or "stand up" for the bullied individual, helping to end the negative interaction. Many people keep silent during a bullying episode, not because they support the bully, but rather they do not want to be involved in the situation. However, by remaining silent, they are, if not implicitly condoning the behavior, creating an environment in which bullying can flourish. It is important, therefore, to train those who are witnessing bullying to come to the aid of those who are being bullied. By doing so, bullies are less likely to act out because they can expect to be challenged on their behavior.

Challenges of Becoming an Upstander

There are a number of reasons why people do not speak up when bullying occurs. Most often people remain silent because they do not want to become a target of bullying themselves. They are concerned that if they try to intervene, the bully will turn his or her attention toward them. Other reasons include not knowing what to say or how to say it, feeling like it is none of their business, expecting someone else to handle it, or not having the physical ability to intervene.

Goals of Upstander Training

The primary goal of upstander training is to convey to members of the community that they each have a responsibility to help thwart bullying behaviors. The training also provides specific intervention strategies and opportunities to practice using the strategies in a group setting.

How to Provide Upstander Training

As part of an ongoing bullying prevention program, gather residents in groups of 30 to 40 people for about an hour of upstander training. Providing light snacks either before or after the meeting will encourage attendance and create a positive atmosphere. Although mandatory meetings have the advantage of making sure that all in the community will receive the training, the forced nature can be seen by some as mimicking bullying and, therefore, might not be the best choice. On the other hand, if residents are left to participate at will, it is likely that the meeting will not be attended by those who need training the most—people who feel it is not their place to intervene in bullying situations.

In cases such as these, encourage everyone to attend and offer an individual invitation to those who would most benefit from the training but might not attend without some encouragement. This reassurance is best offered by someone who has a good relationship with the person. Residents could be asked to champion attendance with their friends and neighbors, or an individual could be encouraged to participate with a comment such as, "Dr. Barbera is hoping to see you there." Other ways to encourage attendance include the chance to participate in a raffle or invitations with a handwritten note.

During the first 10 minutes of the training, define bullying as "intentional, repetitive, aggressive behavior involving an imbalance of power and strength" (Hazelden Foundation, 2008) and describe the cycle of bullying as presented in Figure 7.2. Point out how the lack of intervention by onlookers empowers the bully and increases bullying behaviors. Answer any questions from the group about what does and does not constitute bullying among peers.

During the next 30–45 minutes, divide the larger group into smaller subgroups of four or five. If cliques have formed during the seating process (i.e., friends sitting near each other), consider breaking them up (e.g., ask the participants to count off and have all the "ones" sit together, all the "twos" together, etc.). If residents

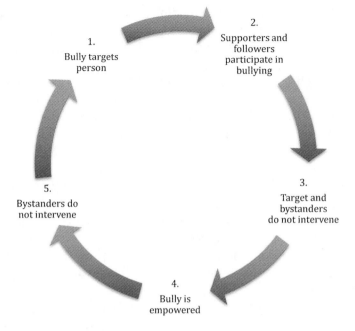

Figure 7.2. The cycle of bullying.

require assistance to move about the room, gather people in small groups from the beginning so that it is not necessary to rearrange the seating.

Then ask each group to choose one person to act as the bully and another person to be the target. As part of this round, ask the other group members to join in and antagonize the bully. Introduce the exercise by saying, "Although bullying is a serious topic, we're going to have some fun with it today." Inject humor into the exercise by asking the bully to harass the volunteer target about something completely outlandish (e.g., teasing the target about the color of his or her shoes). In keeping with the light-hearted tone of the exercise, remind participants that the bullying should be verbal or relational and not physical or aggressive. Maintaining a jocular mood during the training creates an enjoyable atmosphere where camaraderie can flourish among peers who might not have previously engaged with one another. It also sets the tone for the type of community that the exercise hopes to foster: a place where people can work together to solve a common problem and have fun doing it.

Allow the groups about 5 minutes to engage in the role-play, and then stop the exercise and ask participants from several or all of the groups, depending on the time allotted, how they felt about the bullying, being bullied, and being the bullies. A common reaction is a feeling of discomfort about the exercise itself, because most people do not intentionally engage in bullying. Taking the participants out of their comfort zone is part of the exercise so that they can feel more prepared when confronted with bullying in the community.

In the second part of the training, ask the targets and bullies to switch roles. This time, encourage bystanders to stand up to the bully and to try to put a stop to it. Remind the group to be as outlandish in their bullying as possible. After 5 minutes, stop the groups and ask them to share their feelings, reactions, and methods for stopping the bullying. If there is time, ask each subgroup to share how they handled the situation.

There are many ways to stop bullies, and chances are excellent that your participants will have come up with a good variety of techniques, including:

- siding with the target ("I like those shoes!")

- deflecting or changing the subject ("You know, that reminds me of a pair of shoes I saw in the store the other day.")

- using humor (A Chinese elder participating in the exercise told the bully she was eating too much meat, a comment that is associated in Chinese culture with being aggressive: "You need to eat more vegetables!")

- removing the target from the interaction ("I need your help. Can you come with me?")

Other methods of addressing bullying include pointing out the behavior to the bully ("When you say that, you come across as a bully"), or telling a staff member about the interaction.

If your groups have not used many different techniques, take time to have a general discussion about other ways they could have intervened. Wrap up the meeting by encouraging participants to use in the community what they have learned through the upstander training.

Second-Level Intervention:
A Resident Recognition Program

A resident recognition program seeks to encourage positive behaviors among residents. The program clearly outlines what behaviors are considered worthy of acknowledgement and provides rewards that are satisfying to the participants. Just as companies recognize long-time employees, many organizations already acknowledge residents for their long-standing tenure in the community. A successful resident recognition program, however, goes beyond appreciating longevity by using the award ceremony as a teachable moment. By describing specifically what the individual did that was considered notable, others can learn from the behaviors of their peers. For example, an individual might receive an award for the core value of "Caring" because he or she "visited a peer who wasn't feeling well, brought her chicken soup, and cheered her up."

A program such as this has a number of notable benefits, including the following:

- outlines the core values of a community

- describes in detail a behavior that exemplifies a community value

- provides the opportunity for others to learn about what types of behaviors a community considers to be of value

- encourages staff members to be aware of positive interactions between residents and to share them with organization management

- offers a valuable reward to the person being recognized (a certificate and acknowledgement in front of peers)

To adapt and implement this program in a senior community, start by determining the core values of your organization. Because this is an anti-bullying intervention, the values chosen should relate to those that create a caring, friendly community in which bullying behavior is discouraged. Some examples of values include:

- *Welcoming new community members*, which focuses on helping those new to the community feel a part of their new environment by inviting them to meals or activities, being part of a formal "welcoming committee," introducing newcomers to a mutual friend, and so forth. New members of a community are particularly vulnerable to bullying because they have not yet made social connections, and bullies tend to target isolated individuals.

- *Acting as an upstander*, which involves standing up for others against bullying in a variety of ways.

- *Offering encouragement*, whereby peers reach out to each other to support their endeavors, which could range from attending activities to following up on a medical appointment (keeping details private, of course).

- *Being helpful*, which could include assisting a fellow resident with anything from hanging a picture to making a difficult telephone call.

- *Lending support*, such as by bringing a meal to someone who is ill or visiting a fellow resident after the loss of a family member.

Your organization might consider incorporating other positive values, such as showing determination, courage, willpower, or persistence. The characteristics of civility described in Chapter 4 could also be used to encourage positive behaviors among residents.

Choosing Values

For the rewarded values to truly reflect the community, selection should include feedback from the residents. The level of resident involvement depends on the type of organization and the residents' ability to participate. Some organizations with very capable and active residents might find that residents can take the lead in choosing core values, with only minor input from staff or management. Other organizations may find it practical to select a number of values and allow the residents to vote on specifics. A resident committee could also be formed to present recommendations to residents for voting, with input from staff and management as needed. It is also important to consider the number of values selected; five or six values would allow for enough variety to start the program without becoming overwhelming.

Nominating Residents

Allowing residents to nominate one another has two benefits: it allows for more community involvement as well as more eyes to watch for positive interactions. Consider creating a nomination form that elicits information about which value the person is being nominated for and the specifics of why he or she is being nominated. Such a form can also allow nominations to be made anonymously.

It can also be valuable for staff members to nominate residents. Staff nominations can jump-start a recognition program if peer nominations are initially slow in coming. Staff nominations can model for residents how and why to nominate. Staff members can also use the nomination process to "flip the script" on residents who generally exhibit negative behaviors. For example, a resident who is perceived as aloof might be commended for lending a hand to a neighbor, or a quiet, bullied resident might be honored for some unexpected strength or action. Similarly, an individual who tends to bully others might be nominated for a rare show of kindness, which could serve to motivate more kind behaviors.

The Ceremony

One of the most important features of an award ceremony is its sustainability. If the festivities are too elaborate, they are less likely to be maintained and, in turn, might undermine the efforts of those involved. It is far better to add the acknowledgement ceremony to an already-established event than to create a separate event if it is unlikely to be continued. For example, if your organization already holds a monthly birthday event, consider adding on a 15-minute recognition ceremony. Alternatively, some organizations might find a quarterly acknowledgement more sustainable than a monthly occasion. Do what works best for your community.

An organization that is able to commit to a stand-alone ceremony on a regular basis might consider including the following elements:

- Begin with an introduction by a senior staff member who can highlight the importance of the community values and the residents who uphold those values.

- Include a musical performance or other exhibit of talent by residents, such as a photo or craft exhibit, or host a bake sale to benefit the residents or a selected charity.

- Notify residents being rewarded so that they may invite friends and family members.

- Present awards that represent a variety of the community's values.

Rewards

Often the ceremony and acknowledgement itself is enough of a reward for residents. Other options include a framed or unframed certificate, a small bouquet of flowers, a meal of their choice in the dining hall, or a gift certificate to a local establishment. Consider that if the event is special enough, it might be an opportunity for promoting the organization to the larger community. Nearby shops might be willing to contribute their merchandise or gift certificates if the name of their establishment is printed in a program accompanying the event. A local newspaper might cover the festivities, or local high school students might want to lend a hand for some intergenerational fun. Again, determine what is feasible and likely to be maintained over time so there is long-term consistency to the ceremony and acknowledgement.

Third-Level Intervention: Pro-Social Activities

The third level of intervention is based on the concept that people who are busy "doing good" in the world do not have time to engage in bullying behavior. In fact, anecdotal evidence suggests that the level of bullying in communities decreased when residents engaged in pro-social activities. Although reducing bullying was not the goal of the organizations, it was an unanticipated positive side effect of offering pro-social activities to residents. Encouraging pro-social activities within a community is likely to have a positive impact on residents through enhanced self-esteem and reduced symptoms of depression. In addition, the organization may experience benefits such as increased positive visibility within the community and greater occupancy rates.

What Are Pro-Social Activities and Why Offer Them?

A pro-social activity involves resident engagement in an endeavor that is designed to help others outside of the community. Examples include a group of older adults who knit hats for premature babies at a local hospital, raising money for a charity, or making telephone calls or stuffing envelopes for a political campaign.

Often those living in senior communities have many of their lifelong activities taken care of by others, such as keeping a home or taking care of finances. Without these activities and other defining roles, such as wage earner or parent of a young child, older adults can feel a lack of purpose to their lives. In the absence of purpose, depression and boredom can set in. Some people may turn to gossip and other bullying behaviors in order to create excitement, drama, and a sense of activity in their lives. The goals of pro-social activities are to replace negative behaviors with positive enterprises, to keep people busy so there is no time for bullying and to create an environment at odds with bullying behaviors.

Choosing the Activities

Again, the more the residents can be involved in the decision making, the more invested they will be in the process and outcome. Some communities may be able to leave the choice of pro-social activities completely up to the residents. Others may offer residents the ability to vote among several choices. Keep in mind that local charities may offer a community an opportunity to interact with the recipients of their support efforts, such as through a local food bank or animal shelter. Such activities also offer good publicity for senior organizations that may hope to attract new residents from the local community.

Promoting an Activity

For maximum impact in decreasing bullying behaviors, use a pro-social activity as an opportunity to engage as many members of the community as possible, including bullies and the targets of bullying. Engaging a target of bullying in a lifelong skill or connecting him or her with peers through shared activities makes it less likely that the person will be bullied in the future. Bullies tend to seek isolated individuals. Alternatively, engaging a bully in a positive activity reduces the amount of time to bully and allows for successful peer interactions.

As with the resident recognition program ceremony, pro-social activities should be selected with sustainability in mind. Some communities may be able to generate excitement for successive fundraising efforts and include staff and family members in such activities. Other communities will be more successful with a year-long effort focused on a single goal.

Summary

Assessing and reassessing bullying prevention programs is essential regardless of the interventions used. Doing so allows the community to target the areas most in need of modification and to determine whether the techniques used have been successful. Consider beginning with an upstander training program and then add second- and third-level interventions as the programs become regular features of the community.

CHAPTER 8

Empathy Training

~~~~~~

The Different Like Me Culture

Alyse November

What comes to mind when you hear the word *bully*? For most people, the word conjures an image of a child, maybe in middle or high school, picking on another younger or smaller child, teasing him, beating him up, or taking his lunch money. Although bullying among older adults typically does not look like it does among children, it exists and it is no less devastating and harmful. Among older adults, bullying is far more covert and embedded in regular, everyday interactions, such as with the following examples:

- "Hurry up, Harriet. Put your purse on that chair. Here comes June. She has a memory problem, and I can't stand having a conversation with her. She keeps repeating the same story over and over again."

- "Betty, I don't want to invite Sally to the outing next week. She's going to slow us down because of her walker."

This is the face of bullying among older adults, and it is pervasive in 55+ communities, assisted living, independent living, and even community day programs. However, there is very little awareness of this problem among the general population. An Internet search of the term *senior bullying* produces a very limited number of articles on the topic. Even professionals who work with older adults appear unaware that this type of behavior exists. Why is there such a lack of awareness of the social problems regularly faced by older adults? Perhaps it is the ingrained societal myth that most older people tend to keep to themselves. As they near the end of their lives, they are expected to isolate themselves. This myth is not only inaccurate, but also contributes to an acceptance of withdrawal and isolation as somehow natural states of being among older adults. In addition, it prevents insights into the painful consequences of negative social interactions. The truth is, most people move into retirement communities with the expectation of being more socially engaged and less isolated. They anticipate having access to a great many activities and people with whom to interact. Unfortunately, the pervasiveness of bullying among older adults can turn the myth into a reality. People move into a retirement community only to find cliques of men and women who exclude and devalue them. In turn, the targets of this behavior withdraw and isolate themselves, reinforcing and perpetuating the power of the bullies. The section that follows is an example of a program that has been developed to help counter the effects of bullying for older adults.

Appreciating the Reality of Bullying Among Elders

Despite having worked in the mental health field for more than 25 years and having worked primarily with older adults for the past decade, I was similarly unaware of the problem of bullying among older adults. During a lunch with friends who also work with older adults—an attorney in elder law, the owner of a home health agency, and a professional guardian/care manager—the topic of bullying among children came up. I described the very successful bullying prevention program called Different Like Me that I had developed and implemented in the Palm Beach County Public School system. The program focused on preventing bullying by fostering empathy in all students, including the potential bullies, by putting children in the shoes of the target of the bullying to help them feel and understand what it is like to be bullied and helping them to adapt their behavior in a positive manner. The results were astounding. Following the program, participating schools reported a 75% reduction in bullying incidents, making it clear that it was a lack of empathy that contributed to childhood bullying and that if children are taught to think about how their actions impact others, there will be a corresponding reduction in bullying behaviors.

This conversation led to a comparison of children's behaviors and the different, but all-too-similar, behaviors experienced by my lunch mates' older clients. They then told me story after story about the ways some of their older clients were being bullied, belittled, ostracized, and excluded. In an "ah-ha moment," it became apparent that a problem that had been addressed so successfully among children in the Palm Beach County schools was a problem that existed well beyond school, and with similarly devastating effects. The behaviors observed in childhood bullies also exist among older adults, but have transformed into more-subtle, covert behaviors. In other words, bullies do not mature; they just get older.

Unfortunately, very little information on bullying among older adults exists. Therefore, I began interviewing people ages 55 and older, inquiring whether they had witnessed, engaged in, or been the targets of mean-spirited, exclusionary bullying behaviors. Not surprising, the vast majority of people reported that they had witnessed this kind of behavior frequently in their communities, and many admitted that it had happened to them. Few, however, were able or willing to admit that they had engaged in bullying behaviors themselves.

Not only has lack of awareness of bullying among older adults led to an absence of research into the nature and cause of the problem, there is also a dearth of interventions to address it. As a result, I adapted the Different Like Me program to work with older adults, and the Different Like Me Culture: Senior Culture program was born. Senior Culture is a web-based, interactive educational program that focuses on the prevention of bullying by transforming people into sensitive, aware individuals and, ultimately, encouraging their communities to evolve into nurturing, caring, and inclusive environments. Senior Culture offers interactive, web-based educational programming to residents and staff in senior living or senior care organizations to help them understand and effectively manage common issues arising from lack of sensitivity, empathy, and acceptance. The Senior Culture program can be found at www.dlmculture.com.

Piloting the Senior Culture Program

Piloting the Senior Culture program to determine its effectiveness was imperative. The entire lesson series was presented to the residents of two independent living facilities in south Florida over a 4-month period, and included educating them about relationship issues that arise within senior communities as well as fostering the development and use of empathic skills. Participants openly shared stories about how mean some of the residents had been, bullying incidents they had witnessed or in which they were involved, how bullying made them feel intimidated and vulnerable and caused them to withdraw and isolate themselves, and how they felt that the facility administration was not contributing to a solution. As the lessons progressed and participants began to use the empathic skills learned through the program, there were visible, positive transformations in the participants as well as in their interactions. As part of the piloting process, participants completed pre-evaluations that compiled demographic information; examined their knowledge of bullying behaviors; and asked about friendships they had in the facility, how they and others were treated by other residents and staff, and if they had been bullied or witnessed others being bullied. Prior to initiating the pilot program, one facility administrator said: "We desperately need this type of program; some of the residents are so mean to each other. They exclude each other from card games, activities, and socializing in the dining room. It is horrible, and no matter what I do, I can't seem to get them to be nice to one another." An activity director added, "It is like middle school all over again—there is an 'in crowd,' and if you are not part of it, then you are left out." At the conclusion of the pilot program, a post-test was administered to the same residents inquiring about changes in their awareness of bullying, their development of empathy, and the impact on the behavior of those in their community regarding how they view and treat others.

The results of the post-evaluation revealed a very positive impact on the attitudes and behaviors of the participants:

- 100% of the residents reported that they became more sensitive to the needs of others.

- More than 75% felt that they were better able to respond and help others who were the targets of bullying.

- More than 90% reported that they stopped judging others by the way they looked and behaved.

- 70% felt more accepted by their community and found it easier to make and keep new friends.

These results were consistent with those of the original Different Like Me program for school children; pre-and post-tests showed a 75% reduction in bullying behaviors. This suggested that the original hypothesis was correct: a lack of awareness and empathy contributed to bullying behaviors in older adults, just as it had in children. As a result of these promising findings, the Senior Culture program was launched.

Program Production

The Senior Culture program is the first of its kind, and consists of a lesson series aimed at helping older adults and senior care staff to develop empathy and thereby create a positive emotional climate and community culture in which bullying is unacceptable. It is designed to be adaptable and useful in any and every community in which older adults interact. Easily accessed via computer, the lessons are presented in a video format and are accompanied by a written lesson plan and downloadable activities as PDF files. The lessons can be effectively administered by a facilitator without any formal training.

The success of the Senior Culture program is based on many different factors, including the engaging nature of the programming, the use of real-life scenarios, the thought-provoking and interactive activities, and the community-building exercises. The overall objective of the Senior Culture lessons is to foster empathy, the single most important skill necessary in building close relationships, maintaining friendships, and developing strong and caring communities. Without empathy, a community lacks connection, understanding, compassion, and respect. Without empathy, communities often have an overall negative emotional climate and no cohesive culture.

The Senior Culture Lesson Series

Empathy

The concept of empathy is an integral part of the Senior Culture program. Empathy, as mentioned in chapter 5, is by definition the ability to understand and share the feelings of another. Empathy is often explained as the ability to stand in another person's shoes. Individuals who bully are not being empathic, and their interactions become "me" centered. The following example illustrates this phenomenon:

> *Betty:* "Don't look now, here comes Sally using a new walker. Whatever you do, Gladys, don't invite her to the outing at the mall. She will only slow us down."
>
> *Gladys:* "Betty, why are you always so mean to her? Sally is a really nice person."
>
> *Betty:* "You know, Gladys, if you are going to take Sally's side, we might have to exclude you."

Exaggerated? Not really. This is a common scenario in which one resident, Betty, lacks the ability to be empathic. It was all about Betty and how she would be impacted and inconvenienced by Sally's use of a walker, without regard for Sally or Gladys. Empathy, although simple in definition, is a challenging concept for some, which is why the program devotes four lessons to developing it.

The lessons on empathy also teach participants the tools to transform the concept of empathy into feelings, thoughts, and actions. Among many other activities, the first lesson includes a story of moral dilemma in which one character struggles to step outside of her comfort zone and invite a sad, lonely woman into her group with the knowledge that her friends may not approve. The two characters in the story never say a word to each other, but have a strong connection. After the story is read, the participants are encouraged to engage in a discussion about the characters by connecting the story to their own feelings and personal experiences. During the piloting phase of the program, one participant began crying as she told a similar story of exclusion, and everyone in the group embraced her.

Participants are also encouraged to get in touch with their own feelings in learning to be more emphathetic. We all have feelings and emotions related to events and situations, and our responses are based on those feelings. In order to be empathetic, a person must first be able to recognize, understand, and have control over his or her own responses to an event or situation. During one of the pilot programs, a participant, Fran, openly shared that her friend, Sue, recently fractured her hip and was now in a wheelchair. While sitting with her friends in the dining room for dinner, Fran saw Sue being wheeled in. Fran said: "Here comes Sue. Look, she's in a wheelchair. If she thinks she's going to come and sit with us, she should think again. I'm not squeezing all of us in around this little table to fit that big wheelchair. She'll just have to find another table to sit at from now on."

Fran clearly had no qualms about sharing with everyone that she did not want to be inconvenienced by Sue. She did not ask her tablemates for their opinions and did not seem to care about the impact of her attitude on them or Sue. She was not aware that what she was saying was wrong or hurtful because she was so enveloped in her own emotional process. Until Fran is able to recognize and understand her own feelings, she will not be able to develop empathy for others. It was truly amazing to finally witness Fran's transformation after participating in the lesson on empathy. She expressed that she was not angry with Sue; rather, her feelings and behavior were borne out of a desire to avoid facing her own fears of becoming disabled.

The empathy lesson teaches participants that feelings are not right or wrong and that they cannot be controlled. However, the way you act on your feelings and respond to situations can be controlled. Participants complete the lesson with a better understanding of how to recognize and understand their own feelings as well as how the choices they make in responding to situations can affect others.

How Do I Stand in Your Shoes?
How Do I Know How You Feel?

The success of the Senior Culture program can largely be attributed to its ability to help participants feel what it is like to stand in another's shoes, namely that of a person being bullied. Participants feel the effects of bullying through unconventional and nonthreatening methods with the goal of having them understand what it feels like to be teased, excluded, shunned, or talked about, as expressed by Sharon, a participant: "I had no idea how it felt to be left out. I have been so mean to Phyllis since she moved in over a year ago, and now I know how she feels." Sharon sobbed during most of this lesson. Later, she and Phyllis dined together.

With its focus on interactive, experiential learning, this lesson in particular on how to stand in another's shoes has helped many participants find the courage to share their personal stories of how they were being excluded or how they excluded others. After completing this lesson with participants, staff have reported a noticeable improvement in the overall emotional climate of the facility, as residents seemed to be nicer to and more accepting of each other.

Making It Work, Even When It Doesn't

The lesson on making relationships work teaches participants how to make positive connections with almost everyone, even with those with whom it can be very challenging to engage. People may initially "rub you the wrong way," and you choose not to have anything to do with them. Typically, it takes multiple experiences with a person to develop a connection. Relationships take work. As part of this lesson, participants are asked to consider, for example, the following scenario:

> Sally and Betty used to be best friends. They did everything together: shopping, socializing, card games, everything. But recently, Betty's mental state has declined, and Sally is finding it hard to spend time with her. Betty has been diagnosed with Alzheimer's disease and is sometimes challenging to be with. How should Sally handle this situation?

Unfortunately, this is an all-too-real scenario that is played out on a daily basis in senior living and senior care communities. The number of people diagnosed with cognitive loss is growing at an alarming rate, and changes in memory are often why people are excluded and shunned by others. Senior Culture research has shown that memory loss is just one of many challenges that can cause disharmony in relationships. However, just because Betty has Alzheimer's disease does not mean that she cannot experience emotions and recognize she is being excluded. Although Sally does not want to be mean to her friend, she must recognize how she is affected by her friend's disease. Should Sally sacrifice her own needs to make her friend happy, or does she disappoint Betty and exclude her? This question poses a moral and ethical dilemma that is commonly confronted in relationships. This lesson builds on the tools learned in the previous lessons to help participants develop the skills necessary to use empathy in situations where connecting with another person may be challenging.

Let's Be Different

Research on childhood bullying indicates that being perceived as different from others is one of the instigating factors behind being bullied (see Chapter 2). Research done by Senior Culture has shown much the same. A lack of acceptance of other's differences is directly correlated with bullying behaviors and causes people to ridicule, exclude, and talk about their peers. In order to develop a true sense of empathy for one another, one must recognize that differences are just differences, not good or bad, right or wrong, and learn to find a level of acceptance.

The lesson on differences helps to "even the playing field" through role-playing that encourages participants to look at their perceptions of others. It challenges participants to answer questions such as, "What makes your differences better or worse than another's? Who gave you the power to make that decision?" Participants are encouraged to embrace each other's differences and become sensitive to the needs of others. Consider, for example, the following two scenarios:

> "Don't ask Harriet to sit with us at the theater. She shops for most of her clothes in the clearance rack, and nothing matches. I don't want to be seen with her!"

> "Don't look now, but here comes Fred. He's not as sharp as he used to be. Quick, look away when he walks by. Maybe he won't ask us to join in the poker game. I can't stand to play with him; he always makes mistakes."

These scenarios are mild compared to what is actually occurring in senior communities, which is why it is imperative to tackle the issue of differences head on. After completing this lesson, Sally, who made the comments about Harriet's clothing, was able to recognize her own differences and acknowledge that Harriet's choice to shop in a thrift store was no better or worse than her own choices of where to shop. More important, she was able to see the inherent unfairness in excluding someone because of some perceived difference. By recognizing her own differences, Sally also realized that they could potentially make her just as vulnerable to the bullying and exclusion of others. Whether a participant is able to vocalize personal feelings and share experiences is irrelevant. After completing this lesson, each and every participant is able to see what makes them different from others, to recognize the vulnerability inherent in those differences, and to realize the unfairness of using those differences as a justification for bullying.

Bullying

Once bullying has occurred, the damage has already been done. Bullying behaviors can have devastating effects on both targets and bystanders and can trigger depression, anxiety, isolation, loneliness, and even suicide. Thus, prevention is the only long-term, sustainable solution to combat this problem. The previous lessons begin the process of bullying prevention by teaching empathy, making positive connections, and normalizing differences. The lesson on bullying teaches participants about bullying behaviors, such as in the following scenario:

> Harry was walking by the exercise room and saw Mary exercising along with some of the other community residents. "Keep up the exercise, Mary. You're still fat."

People like Harry reside in every senior community. Is Harry a bully? Did he engage in bullying behavior? Harry's example of bullying is typical as well as quite overt. Many other instances of bullying, however, are much more covert. For example, Susan related a story that she never told anyone before. She reported that when she and her husband first moved into their community, they went to the dining room for breakfast. They walked over to a table that had two empty seats and were told that those seats were taken. They then walked over to another table that had empty seats and were told that they could not sit there either. The couple then took their trays upstairs to their room and never returned to the dining room again for breakfast, even 3 years later.

Often, the targets of bullying feel powerless and suffer in silence. Many residents explain this phenomenon with statements such as "We are old and want to live the rest of our lives in peace." "We feel vulnerable and scared that things will get worse." "It's easier to avoid [the bullies] than it is to try to change things."

The lesson on bullying begins to take participants on an interactive journey to learn more about senior bullying behaviors. Three other lessons in the program series further engage participants by teaching them how to successfully manage situations that involve bullying behaviors, whether as a bystander, through peer pressure, or by coming into direct contact with a bully. The lesson activities provide participants with the skills to think quickly on their feet when faced with a challenging bullying situation.

The Powerful Bystander

Because bullying does not occur within a vacuum involving only the bully and the target, the Senior Culture program includes a lesson on being an active bystander. Research on childhood bullying has shown that bystanders can be highly instrumental in preventing a bullying incident. When a bystander intervenes, he or she can stop an incident that involves bullying within 10 seconds more than 50% of the time (Hawkins, Pepler, & Craig, 2001). Even though most bystanders report that they do not like to witness bullying, fewer than 20% try to stop it. Furthermore, statistics show that 85% of bullying incidents are witnessed by bystanders. Then, why do these witnesses not step in and help the target? The vast majority of older adults polled suggested that a lack of understanding and knowledge of how to intervene, as well as a fear of becoming the target, were the reasons for their inaction. During this lesson, one of the participants, Gail, described a situation in which she saw Grace bullying another resident:

> "I'm sick and tired of hearing you bellyache about your problems! We as a group are done with you, and you're no longer welcome to join us for anything! Right, ladies? Tell Lois how we're tired of hearing her complain. Good luck finding a new set of friends. I'm going to tell everyone about how you whine and complain all the time. No one will be your friend."

Gail was afraid that if she stepped in and stood up to Grace, then Grace would in turn bully her. After completing the training, however, Gail reported that she had witnessed Grace bullying another person. She explained that she used a technique she had learned in the lesson on being an active bystander, and it worked! Specifically, when she witnessed Grace bullying her friend Harriet, Gail was able to safely remove Harriet from the situation by politely interrupting Grace and asking Harriet for her help in an urgent matter. Harriet accepted Gail's request for help and, as the two of them walked away, Gail provided emotional support to Harriet and suggested that she stay away from Grace. Gail felt so empowered and was happy she could help her friend.

Because of the risks involved in intervening, this lesson teaches the skills necessary for participants to become active, positive bystanders without putting themselves in harm's way.

Senior Culture research has shown that bystanders play a huge role in stopping bullies in their tracks. The organization is, therefore, engaged in a future development project to create a three- to five-part series that focuses solely on empowering the bystander.

Pressuring Peers

Peer pressure is another major issue that affects relationships as well as the overall emotional climate of a community. The pressure to conform and the feeling that you are stuck having to choose between what you want to do and what someone else is pressuring you to do can be very powerful and difficult to deal with. Although not all peer pressure is harmful, when it has negative implications and resembles bullying, it can cause a social situation to implode. Negative peer pressure, very much like bullying, may be expressed openly: "No, don't invite Betty to dinner tonight; she's not like us." More frequently, however, it is delivered through subtle, silent signals:

> Gloria explained that she is part of a group of women in the community. She described herself as the person who does not get noticed among some of the stronger personalities of the group. Gloria went on to say that she feels as if she never has a voice. She typically goes along with what all of the others say and do. Otherwise, she fears she will be excluded from the group. Gloria does not feel that some of the more boisterous members of the group are nice or fair toward others. In fact, "they are downright mean. They told me that if I sat next to Betty on the upcoming trip to the casino, they wouldn't talk to me the whole time we were there. They are bossy and mean. I feel like I'm back in middle school! Heck, this is even worse than middle school because I'm trapped in this residence for the remainder of my life. When I was in school, at least I could go home where no one bullied me and there was no peer pressure. I really thought that it wouldn't be like this here."

As part of this lesson, many of the other program participants began to open up and share with the group their experiences with peer pressure. As the lesson continued, the participants learned how to address and manage peer pressure by engaging in an activity called "Stuck in the Middle," which encourages independence within a group by allowing each person to make decisions for him- or herself, even if it goes against the group's thinking. As a wonderful ending to this lesson, the participants started a "No Peer Pressure" campaign, encouraging all residents to make decisions for themselves about how they would interact with each other and not allow others to pressure them.

Head On

Conflict is a naturally occurring and unavoidable part of a relationship. The lesson on how to successfully manage conflict teaches participants to see the process as a need for change as well as an opportunity for growth and improved communication. When people come together, conflict is bound to occur. Saving seats in the dining room, not allowing someone to join in on a game of Mah Jong, and making negative remarks about others are all opportunities for conflict to arise. Managing conflict can be quite challenging and, typically, most people do not do it very well:

> Bess explained that one of her friends had recently become a widow and, as a result, had been keeping to herself. Despite numerous invitations, this woman constantly turned down Bess' invitations. Bess was feeling very sad at losing this friendship and chose to speak with her group of friends to get their support. Unfortunately, May, one of the more outspoken members of this group, expressed to Bess that she was "sick and tired of hearing about this problem, and if you continue to talk about it, consider yourself out of this group."

Bullying, by nature, creates conflict, and the lesson on conflict resolution teaches participants simple techniques to consider the various perspectives of those involved, understand their thoughts and feelings, and develop strategies for resolving the dispute in a manner that is acceptable to everyone involved. In the May and Bess situation, the particpants felt that it would be helpful to explain to May that Bess was feeling lonely and rejected and that trying to share those feelings with her friends was her way of seeking support at a difficult time. They felt that May should be encouraged to be more understanding and supportive of Bess versus threatening to exclude Bess from the group by making her feel as though she was bringing the issue up over and over again.

Research through Senior Culture has shown that using participants' own experiences helps them to understand and successfully use the concepts they learn through the training in a more meaningful way. It is important, therefore, that program administrators encourage participants to discuss their own personal stories and experiences to guide this lesson's activities. The pilot program showed that participants were better able to retain and use the techniques and information they had learned by sharing their own experiences. Managing conflict is no easy task, but when done successfully, the result is well worth the time and effort.

Use It or Lose It!

Teaching older adults the skills to deal with bullying is one goal, but having them apply those skills consistently is the key to bringing about change. The strategies and tools learned through the Senior Culture program are not meant to be used only for the hour in which the participants are actively engaged. Rather, they should be used to create a sustainable, positive emotional climate that is clearly visible to all who enter the community. When piloting the program, administration was invited to attend the lesson on "use it or lose it" to discuss how to sustain the program by, for example, forming a committee or holding a monthly meeting for staff, administration, and residents to come together to discuss how to create a sensitive, cooperative community.

Top Down or Bottom Up?

Staff and administrators participate in the Senior Culture programming alongside residents. Both groups really need to understand the issue of bullying from their own perpectives to create and sustain a healthy emotional climate within the community. Because research on bullying among older adults is so limited, best current practices are based on an understanding of the emotional safety of children and the correlation of a proactive, involved administration. A school is a type of community in which people interact, the same as a senior residence is a community. If an educator or principal does not address bullying behavior at the administrative level, are they not tacitly condoning it? An attitude of "not my concern" on the part of teachers and administration sends a message to students that bullying behavior is acceptable, thereby creating an emotionally unsafe atmosphere for students. The same goes for bullying among older adults. The residence administrator, as well as nurses, aides, and dining room staff, must all support the mission of building a caring, empathic community in which bullying is not tolerated.

Bullying among older adults has largely gone unnoticed and been unaddressed because there was nothing available to educate staff and administrators in senior communities. Senior Culture programming includes a lesson series specifically for staff and administration so that they, too, can be actively engaged in creating a positive emotional climate in which bullying is unacceptable.

Staff Lesson Series

Consisting of four parts, the lesson series for staff and administrators provides continuing education credits to most participants. The sequence of the lessons has been carefully designed to ensure success. The first lesson addresses personal issues that staff and administrators bring to the workplace, as well as how their own social and cultural differences affect their ability to foster a positive emotional climate within the senior community. It also addresses bullying behavior engaged in by the staff themselves. Senior Culture research has found a lack of awareness about what staff bullying behavior looks like, indicating a strong need for education on the topic.

Consider the following scenario:

> The alarm rings. Sam gets out of bed and begins to get himself ready for work. He then remembers that he had a horrible argument with his wife last night and is dreading walking into the kitchen for breakfast and hearing more of his wife's complaints about what he is not doing right. Unfortunately, he has no choice. As predicted, Sam's wife continues the argument from last night,

causing Sam to leave the house feeling angry and frustrated. Sam arrives at Happy Home Residence on time and ready for work. Or was he? Immediately, his boss tells Sam that Mrs. B in room 201 is irate because no one came to fix the lock on her door as promised yesterday. Sam gathers up his tools and takes the elevator to the second floor, all the while thinking about the arguments he had with his wife. He knocks on Mrs. B's door, and, not unlike the conversation she had with Sam's boss earlier that morning, Mrs. B begins to yell and scream at Sam, telling him how disappointed she is with the service provided at Happy Home Residence. She also says that she is going to call her daughter to tell her that she wants to move out. Having been yelled at by his wife that morning, Sam has brought all of his emotional baggage with him to work. Now he is being yelled at by Mrs. B. Frustrations compounded, Sam yells right back at Mrs. B and tells her that she is an angry, mean old lady and she should move out. He also tells her that Happy Home Residence would be a much better place if she were to leave. Mrs. B then throws Sam out of her unit and immediately calls the administrator to complain. There was nothing the administrator could say to fix the situation; the damage had already been done. Mrs. B eventually moved out.

This, unfortunately, is one of many true stories. After completing this particular lesson, however, positive transformations in the overall emotional climate of the residence begin to improve. In addition, this lesson provides a forum for administrators to assist or encourage employees to seek out professional guidance and support to resolve major personal problems.

It is also important for staff to recognize bullying behaviors in residents, as in the following example:

Paula and John, part of the dining room staff, are told about Kim, a resident who feels that some of the other residents get special treatment in the dining room. She feels that these "special" residents get the best seats, hot food, and sometimes a meal choice that is not on the menu. Kim has also said that she feels ignored when she needs more water or salt and sometimes waits for 30 minutes to be seated, even when there is an open chair. Are these behaviors recognized as bullying behaviors on the part of the staff? Are they using their power to manipulate a situation? Kim is bullied by some of the residents in the home and is frequently excluded by them. She has reported that staff members have witnessed this behavior and done nothing about it.

This lesson provides staff and administration with "real-life" examples of bullying that they can actively identify with as well as adapt to many other situations. One of the first steps to change is awareness; once you clearly see the situation, prevention is possible.

Not every bullying situation is preventable, which is why the Senior Culture programming devotes an entire staff/administration lesson to conflict resolution. This lesson provides hands-on techniques for assessment, reporting, and mediation skills. Once again, the lessons use real-life scenarios to address conflict between residents, staff, and staff and residents. The program uses congruent climate techniques (CCT) to help staff and administrators create a positive emotional climate in their workplace. Congruent, by definition, is to be "in agreement or harmony." A congruent climate is a community in which everyone is in agreement or in harmony. Consider the following scenario:

> The recreational director is having a challenging day. His kids called and told him they will not be coming to visit him for the holidays, and he is feeling rejected and lonely. Now he has to gather 50 residents and get them organized and on a bus in less than an hour or they will be late for a theater performance. He makes an announcement over the loudspeaker telling all who will be attending the show to meet in the lobby. Feeling very stressed, he takes a head count and only counts 42 people. He does a recount and once again comes up with 42. He screams out to the crowd, "Who is missing?!" "We're going to be late. "It's Betty and her gang again, isn't it?" he demands angrily. "She's always late, and so is her group of friends. I'm sick of this," he says. Residents who witness this outburst begin to chime in about Betty and her group: "We should leave her here." "Yeah, it would serve her right." "I don't like her anyway and would be happier if she wasn't with us."

A very negative emotional climate has emerged from this group, and it all began with one staff member, the one who should be creating a positive emotional climate, the one who should mediate conflict, not create it. Research shows it can take at least 20 minutes to calm people down from an emotional situation once it has begun. In fact, agitation can last all day, creating a negative cycle in the overall emotional climate of the residence. Senior Culture programming teaches staff and administrators how to use congruent climate techniques as a means of interacting and responding to residents to ensure that they are creating and maintaining a positive emotional state for all residents throughout the course of the day. Using the techniques can reduce symptoms of aggression, agitation, frustration, and irritability and on the part of staff and encourages staff to be responsible for and aware of the emotional climate they create.

Summary

No one age group is immune to the impact of bullying behaviors, and everyone should have access to prevention support and assistance in dealing with this devastating problem. Awareness is the first step toward change. The Senior Culture program not only fosters awareness, but provides a framework for education and intervention to reduce bullying behaviors, empower bystanders, and create more empathetic, cooperative, sensitive, and welcoming communities. Chapter 9 discusses ways to address bullying among older adults by fostering an emotional climate throughout the care community that supports social wellness.

CHAPTER 9

Social Wellness Initiatives to Reduce Bullying Among Older Adults

Katherine Parker Cardinal

To address the problem of bullying among older adults, everyone involved in elder care, from directors of nursing to transportation staff, needs to be educated and trained on the issue and must work together within senior communities to combat it. One of the main messages from the first White House Conference on Bullying Prevention in 2011 is that bullying is a form of abuse that can result in depression, anxiety, and other serious health consequences (Shepherd, 2011). This chapter offers information for aging services professionals for implementing organization-wide cultural changes to address bullying among older adults by fostering a better emotional climate in support of social wellness. This chapter does not address social aggression or bullying related to any kind of physical violence that requires mandated reporting, nor does it advise on illegal harassment and discrimination. In addition, a different approach is required for residents with diagnosed forms of dementia or mental illness. Managers must oversee and train staff on these distinctions and handle these matters with clinical expertise.

Experts in the field see an increased need for senior housing staff to understand bullying as a phenomenon. Workers must be able to define, recognize, and realize the importance of bullying intervention and prevention (R. Bonifas, personal communication, September 29, 2015). If the hurtful behavior of bullies goes unchecked or is rewarded, even inadvertently, over time they (and their supporters) gain more license and power. The environment, in turn, increasingly becomes fertile ground for social aggression. Bullying behaviors are projected to become more widespread as baby boomers continue to move into senior housing communities (Barbera, 2015).

Studies of social aggression show that organization-wide structures that convey and support messages of civility make it difficult for bullies to gain the social support necessary to do harm (Berger, 2007; Workplace Bullying Institute, 2014). In fact, most researchers who study bullying view changes in the environment as the key to reducing bullying (Barbera, 2015; Olweus Bullying Prevention Program, 2015; Wiseman, 2001). The "zero tolerance" policies of fully eliminating bullying have, at least in schools, been replaced by more practical and preventive approaches based on a clearer understanding of how to reduce incidents of bullying (Berger, 2007). This shift is a result of 40 years of study begun in the 1970s by Dan Olweus, father of school bullying research. His work, and that of others who have followed, can inform senior housing administrators in need of a new framework for preventing social aggression.

Despite the need, anti-bullying training is not formally incorporated into most senior service organizations today. Staff may lack the knowledge and skills to prevent and intervene in social aggression among residents. A simultaneous problem of bullying among healthcare workers also presents obstacles (Briles, 2009). The organization-wide goal is to raise awareness of the benefits of promoting a culture of civility to create an environment where social wellness is a priority in every aspect of community life. As a first step, an organization's leadership and middle management need to understand and learn how to address bullying among older adults. The organization will ultimately need to be unified in an ongoing commitment to implement civility programming for residents and will need to craft policy and approaches to suit their community's specific needs.

Organization-Wide Culture Change

As healthcare workers and aging services professionals, we are responsible for supporting the whole individual to be optimally "well" in every regard. Older adults must live in an environment of social wellness to be emotionally healthy. When bullying incidents occur among residents, well-meaning managers often respond by bringing in experts to troubleshoot and "fix" the problem. Unfortunately, piecemeal efforts and one-time trainings on bullying and social aggression may backfire and are often not enough. When bullying problems become rampant, ongoing consult with professionals is best, and in certain cases an organizational overhaul in terms of culture change is necessary. Staff on any level can do damage and make matters worse by stepping in with single pieces of information from individual trainings. Targets can become even more vulnerable and bullies may be unintentionally empowered. Focusing efforts on how to make the whole community a place where people treat one another with dignity is best. Yet all staff must be trained to identify bullying and learn the importance of reaching out early on to supervisors, skilled social workers, and psychotherapists.

An understanding of how social or relational bullying operates, within the context of the social system that supports it, is essential for everyone throughout the organization, but particularly for staff at the top. Only then, with management's full support, can intervention strategies be implemented by frontline staff who most often are the ones who witness bullying and who interact with residents the most on a daily basis. If supervisors do not have a working knowledge of how bullying occurs within a social system, frontline staff will not be able to rely on them in critical moments. Organization-wide lack of clarity regarding definitions of bullying undermines all social wellness efforts. The entire staff must work as a unified team to effect change.

A key study in the Netherlands titled "Resident-to-Resident Relational Aggression and Subjective Well-being in Assisted Living Facilities" revealed a critical finding regarding nursing staffs' understanding of bullying and misperceptions of residents' experiences of emotional distress caused by social aggression (Trompetter, Scholte, & Westerhof, 2011). The following is a list of the questions posed to residents in the study. Participants assigned numbers to each statement ranking the items from "0" for "never occurring" to "4" for "occurring several times per week":

1. Some of the other residents ignore me on purpose and do not greet me when I see them in the corridors or dining room.

2. I notice that rumors and gossip are spread about me by other residents.

3. I am teased in a hurtful way repeatedly by one or more other residents.

4. When I talk to a group of co-residents, some people do not talk to me or ignore me on purpose.

5. There are residents who make fun of me behind my back.

6. Some people do not sit at my table on purpose, because they avoid me.

7. There are residents who seem to want other residents to dislike me and/or stop having contact with me.

8. Some residents ask me in an unfriendly manner why I live in the facility.

9. I am not allowed to join a group of co-residents, even if I treat them in a friendly way.

10. I am excluded from activities in the home (such as playing cards or knitting) by other residents.

11. Co-residents criticize me behind my back.

The findings revealed that "nurse reports of relational aggression were not related to any of the measures of residents' subjective well-being." The researchers concluded that "apparently nurses have difficulty discerning incidences of aggression that are perceived as hurtful by residents" (Trompetter, 2011 p. 65). The difference between what nurses perceived and what residents experienced differed greatly among facilities. When the researchers attempted to explain why nurses' perceptions of residents' experiences were incorrect, they posed two possible scenarios: the "use of indirect aggression tactics by older adults" and/or the "non-transparency of groups of residents, making systematic relational aggression hard to detect for nurses" (Trompetter, 2011, p. 65). In part, without being able to clearly identify friendship hierarchies and power relationships among residents within and between friend groups, nursing staff is potentially at a loss for identifying a bully and his or her supporters. This phenomenon appears to be just like social bullying in female adolescent peer groups, where it is often a challenge to decipher who the main aggressor is. (Underwood, 2003) To make matters worse, bullies, despite myths that they are unlikeable, are often attractive and popular individuals. Charm may cloak bullying tendencies in the presence of those with the power to disapprove, judge, or induce a feeling of shame. The study clearly shows the need for staff to evaluate residents' emotional supports and friendship dynamics, or lack thereof, as critical data in identifying social aggression. Subtle forms of isolation and exclusion are both difficult to detect and undo. Senior staff members need to rely on and develop trust with frontline staff most apt to see and report red-flag behaviors, as they will ultimately be enlisted to help reshape group dynamics over time as part of their daily interactions with residents.

When organization leaders are at a loss because they do not witness bullying directly, outside consultants can be helpful in objectively directing staff on ways to dismantle bullying situations. "Hotspots" for bullying, such as dining rooms and activity areas, can be particularly challenging. Changing protocol in these locations may reduce bullying opportunities, according to Alyse November, a social worker and senior advocate. For example, eliminating the practice of saving seats in dining areas, as well as including more staff in residents' activities (who could intervene after proper training), would be helpful (A. November, personal communication, April 13, 2015).

Preventive approaches often do more to foster civility than punitive measures for bullies. Research and experience from school populations, for example, have found that zero tolerance policies may have unintended adverse effects, including driving down reporting (www.stopbullying.gov, 2015). Bullies may also become more adept at concealing their behavior. According to Martin Donlan, an attorney who works on behalf of assisted living and skilled nursing facilities, it would be difficult to enforce zero tolerance in senior housing given older adults' legal rights. For this reason, he suggests it is best to use preventive approaches, such as civility training (M. Donlan, personal communication, May 1, 2015).

Promoting a Culture of Civility and Social Wellness

Even though clarifying what constitutes bullying is necessary for all staff to understand and address the issue, older adults themselves have expressed that it may be more effective to hear an anti-bullying message within a positive framework. In fact, use of the word *bully* with older adults is often met with resistance. A study in the Netherlands found that despite the fact that behaviors explored were consistent with definitions of bullying, older adults emphatically rejected the term *bullying*, arguing that only children are "bullies" (Trompetter et al., 2011). Promoting anti-bullying programs within a positive framework may, therefore, be more effective with older adults. For example, using terms such as *civility, social wellness*, and *caring community* removes the shame associated with bullying and emphasizes the ultimate goals. Developing a positive narrative may also enable managers to more easily engage staff members in the process of change.

Traditionally, social workers have handled social challenges among older adults in senior living environments, just as school guidance counselors handle such challenges among children. However, the trend in schools today is to train all teachers and paraprofessionals to engage in daily efforts to improve social wellness and thereby reduce bullying (Berger, 2007). Gerontologists are hoping a similar approach will reduce incidents of bullying among older adults by training frontline staff to address social challenges among residents. Nurses and personal care aides need structure and support from the organization to take ownership over the social environment to make it a safer place for everyone.

Here are some questions that may reveal potential problems within the social system related to bullying:

- Are nurses and personal care aides with less social power afraid to stand up to residents who bully because they fear becoming targets of bullying themselves?

- Does a bully escape direct involvement by enlisting unsuspecting staff or other residents against his or her target, acting behind the scenes to shun, exclude, or spread rumors or mistruths?

- Does a bully's social rank, financial status, or perceived popularity dissuade bystanders from showing disapproval?

- Are two or more individuals operating together to bully another faction of weaker, more vulnerable individuals?

- Can defenders of the target gather enough influence in the social hierarchy to effectively confront the bully?

- Do the managers know enough about the situation to disempower a bully (or group of bullies) without harming others in the social system?

Although there is no single-best, evidence-based anti-bullying program to use within a senior housing community or senior center, pilot programs are being developed by clinicians and researchers and are in need of funding. Incorporating multi-department staff civility training is necessary for organization-wide social wellness.

Embracing Diversity

Widely known for her expertise on school bullying, cliques, and social hierarchies, best-selling author Rosalind Wiseman advises school administrators, parents, and children around the world. An internationally recognized researcher on children, parenting, bullying, social justice, and ethical leadership, Wiseman serves as an advisor to the U.S. Department of Health and Human Services. Her work, together with anecdotal evidence from interviews with aging services professionals and educators, highlights the need for inclusion and diversity training as part of a community's social wellness endeavor. Wiseman believes that most incidents of bullying combine intolerance of others' differences with abuse of power, such as nurses and personal care aides who have had the experience of being mistreated and rejected by those in their care based on the color their skin. Individuals aligned with any marginalized group are also at risk of becoming targets.

The following true story told by a director in a senior community illustrates the need for diversity programming for staff and residents:

> A woman nursing home resident who had been fully accepted by her peers eventually made the decision to identify herself as a lesbian to her friends. For years, her friends had thought of her as heterosexual. The staff began to notice changes in her demeanor. She began to isolate herself and show signs of depression. Staff initially thought that the changes were due to a new diagnosis of Parkinson's disease and the symptoms associated with that. Eventually, however, staff recognized that the woman's friends began to reject her based on her newly disclosed sexual orientation. They refused to let her play bingo with them anymore. They would no longer let her join them for meals.

Wiseman acknowledges that people gravitate toward those with similar interests and backgrounds and tend to cluster in groups with respect to gender, class, and ethnicity, among other variables. However, when a group colludes to reject individuals from a gathering that is intended to include everyone, then bullying is occurring (Rosalind Wiseman, April 9, 2015, Lecture at Avon High School, Avon, CT).

Unspoken discrimination underlies most social aggression. Dr. Margaret Cruikshank has explored the concerns of the current generation of older adults who fear isolation based on sexual orientation. Cruikshank writes, "lesbians now in their seventies and older differ significantly from a younger cohort, because being known as gay or lesbian was far riskier than it is today and sometimes led to loss of jobs and housing, loss of child custody, banishment from churches, and verbal and physical attacks" (Cruikshank, 2013, p. 122). A 2009 article published in the *Harvard Journal of Law and Gender* on equity and aging explores the challenges lesbian, gay, bisexual, transgender, and questioning (LGBTQ) individuals face regarding emotional security and a sense of belonging as older adults:

> [LGBT elders] encounter hostility and prejudice on the part of health care providers and feel silenced in institutional settings, such as assisted living facilities and nursing homes. At a time when LGBT individuals enjoy an unprecedented degree of social acceptance and legal protection, our LGBT elders are aging—and dying—alone and invisible, and are often denied the basic dignity of being able to share their memories of a life well lived without fear of rejection and reprisal." (Knauer, 2009, p. 304)

Nursing homes, assisted living facilities, and other senior communal settings need programs for both workers and residents that teach and encourage them to embrace diversity to avoid unspoken, and spoken, discrimination, which is often the root of bullying. Programs also need to encourage people in the community to embrace differences in positive ways. Integrating cultural traditions using food, celebrations, books, and film helps bind residents and staff in universal human experiences.

In September 2015, a public high school in the northeastern United States made the local news when anti-Semitic graffiti was found on school property. The principal, Andrew O'Brien, reacted swiftly and strongly to the damage done by students toward their peers. His response, which was supported by the board of education and teachers, highlighted that the students' actions were in opposition to everything the school stood for in terms of inclusion and dignity for every student. His main message was that such actions lay the foundation for creating an environment where bullying can take root. O'Brien responded with an organization-wide approach and took it a step further into the community by distributing via email a letter to the parents of children at all grade levels. The letter demonstrates a progressive mindset of excellence in leadership and the spirit of an organization-wide effort and system-based solution. The letter, in part, is reprinted here:

> No one in our community should be made to feel that they are any less worthy or important based on their race, religion, sexual orientation, or mental or physical abilities. Whenever a community is confronted with ignorance such as this, it is incumbent on the members of that community to work together to address it. Vincent F. Rocchio, author and filmmaker, said that "Racism is something that people can transcend through friendship." Let your friends know that racist comments or jokes aren't cool, funny, or okay. If you see or hear [discriminatory comments] that make you uncomfortable, speak out against it. . . . Get to know people from different groups and step outside of your comfort zone; you will be enriched by their differences, culture, food, music, art, history, and traditions. You will also find that people are very much like you, with dreams, challenges, hopes, and aspirations, as well as with a desire for friendship and the need to be accepted.
>
> This year I will be working with students and staff members to increase our awareness and understanding of the value of diversity within our school community, and I look forward to your help in that endeavor. This is our school and we all deserve to feel safe and respected. . . . I am engaging with our faculty and our student leaders to process what has happened and to plan for future events and programming that will celebrate the diversity of our school. . . . Everyone in our school community needs to feel the same level of respect and belonging; we will not tolerate the actions or words of those who seek to divide us.

Incorporating this spirit of embracing diversity into civility training will go a long way toward promoting a culture of dignity in
senior communities.

The Role of Organizational Leadership in Addressing Bullying Among Older Adults

In creating an emotionally safe environment, aging services
professionals who have social rank and financial power are
essential within an organization in influencing the norms of
civility. Senior housing administrators either may not believe
or may easily dismiss reports of bullying. In these instances,
it may be helpful for colleagues to convince senior staff of the
seriousness of the problem by tracking incidents and gathering anecdotal evidence that shows the nature and effects of
bullying (e.g., see Chapter 4). Be cautious when sharing information, remembering to maintain resident privacy rights. Timing is essential; proper intervention is important, especially
in the early stages of bullying. As mentioned earlier, bullying
behaviors followed by inaction may actually encourage further
bullying (Berger, 2007).

One easily overlooked obstacle in creating an emotionally
safe environment is organization leaders who themselves engage
in social aggression. Leaders with take-charge styles may commonly be rewarded for possessing qualities of strength. However,
if they ever cross over, even occasionally, into actual aggression,
they will quickly lose influence over others. This is also true of
leaders who inadvertently align themselves with bullies over the
larger group and thereby put the norms of civility at risk for everyone. Intelligent leaders who learn about the hallmarks of bullying
will naturally discover their own blind spots, seek counsel, and
become more effective through personal growth. When deliver-
ing a message on the topic of social wellness, their actions will
be consistent with their message, and this authenticity may yield
greater results.

In *The Heart of Change: Real-Life Stories of How People
Change Their Organizations*, Kotter and Cohen (2002) suggest
that leaders, "will have to attack the sturdy silos and difficult pol-
itics . . . in order to create a twenty-first-century organization"
(Kotter and Cohen, 2002). Thus, not only do leaders need to be

fully educated about bullying, they also need to be experts on how to inspire others to effect change. Combining the power of leadership with the ability to inspire others to promote civility is the key to improving organization-wide social wellness, as shown in the following example:

> Diana Benson, service coordinator for an 80-resident HUD housing complex in Ohio with independent older adults as well as those with physical disabilities, has been working on increasing compassion and reducing fear among residents in her building. A couple of years ago, she set out on a mission to improve the spirit in the building. Having worked in social services for 30 years, Benson felt that certain residents were fearful of not getting their needs met. She felt they were being overly aggressive toward one another with the goal of "jockeying into position to access scarce services and resources."
>
> Benson felt compelled to develop her own program to help residents in meeting their needs because she was discouraged by how poorly the residents treated one another. There were various cliques. One group of seven women was at the top of the social hierarchy. "The group would come walking down the hall, and everybody moved out of the way," Benson reported. The "queen bee" of the clique would tell lies about other residents that would cause others to avoid them. She mocked a person with poor hygiene, would say incredibly mean things, and called people awful names behind their backs. Other residents allowed the behavior, and some joined in by laughing. The effect of this social bullying was damaging for many residents. On her own time, Benson figured out how she could change some of the group dynamics. She read the work of Dr. P.M. Forni at Johns Hopkins University on civility. She also took ideas and information from The Civility Project in Duluth, Minnesota. Benson said at first, "I began plastering kindness quotes on the walls all around the building. People started asking me what I was up to and I didn't tell them." Once she had gathered enough information from what was already known about bullying and civility, she developed her own educational program. She did not identify any bullies and even avoided the truth with people who asked her if they were culprits.
>
> Benson said it was at least 6 months before she saw any changes. However, after 2 years she reported that the destructive cliques were gone. Other positives came out of Benson's programming. She and the residents developed a bartering system

whereby people offered services as a way of getting some of their needs met from others in the building. People now cook meals for one another, provide rides to appointments, or help in other ways with tasks someone may have difficulty with or is no longer able to do. "It's all about meeting the underlying needs, inclusion, and just being civil to one another," Benson concluded.

It is important for leaders to realize that they cannot implement programming without professional guidance and ample support. The proper mindset along with adequate resources to fund and support civility initiatives are necessary in order to bring about change. Along with financial commitment, leaders must model civility in all of their interactions, as well as inspire all levels of the organization to support the social wellness of everyone in the community. Social wellness is a foundational element upon which to build programs and policy in senior housing and elder services for current and future generations.

Summary

This chapter outlines from a macro view how senior housing and senior care managers and leaders can make essential changes to support a healthy social climate. Investing in solutions that address the root causes of bullying is critical to long-term management of the problem. Some research suggests that verbal and social aggression can be precursors to physical aggression. This potential correlation is important to explore and supports the need for further funding and research.

Once on the path of civility as part of culture change, there is no real end to learning, growth, and improvement. The wisdom and practice of social wellness is a hallmark feature of communities that uphold high standards of excellence with regard to the dignity of their members. How *all* members of the community are treated—no matter their social status, seniority in the community, or financial power—is a litmus test of sorts for a community's social wellness. Dignity must be available to anyone who joins a community from day one (Rosalind Wiseman, April 9, 2015, lecture at Avon High School, Avon, CT).

Dr. Beth Gershuny, a psychologist at the Izlind Integrative Wellness Center and Institute, believes bullying to be a form of interpersonal trauma because it calls into question the integrity of one's sense of self and shatters the core sense of self as a valuable being. To be bullied is to be devalued, which is a form of emotional assault. Everyone in a bullying situation, even the bully, needs help (B. Gershuny, personal communication, March 4, 2016). We need to provide older adults emotionally healthy living environments that offer adequate mental health supports for the targets of bullying, bullies, and those who witnesses bullying, including staff. We must also galvanize the aging services industry around the important issue of bullying and support research and pilot programs that can lead to the development of evidence-based interventions and programming.

CHAPTER 10

Future Directions

Policy Imperatives to Address Bullying
Among Older Adults

Alyse November
Stephanie Langer

Bullying exists anywhere people gather. It is seen often in the work place and in social organizations. Unlike children, society expects adults to be able to address bullying independently and without the need for systematic intervention or prevention. However, older adults are often not equipped to handle bullying situations when they arise. Surveys have shown that most do not speak up for themselves due to fear of retaliation. Rather, they isolate themselves in order to avoid the bully. As our population ages, there is a concentrated number of people living and socializing in senior care communities and community-based senior services centers, and research shows that bullying in these settings is on the rise. The laws are not moving fast enough to keep up with this new and growing problem. There must be a systematic response to bullying among older adults, including anti-bullying legislation. This chapter provides a model for crafting such legislation for older adults using existing laws that address bullying among children as a starting point.

Scope of the Problem

The fastest growing segment of America's population consists of those age 85 and older (National Center on Elder Abuse,

Administration on Aging). In 2010, there were 5.8 million people age 85 or older (U.S. Census Bureau, 2008). By 2050, it is projected there will be 19 million, and people age 65 and older are expected to comprise 20% of the total U.S. population (U.S. Census Bureau, 2010). With more people living longer, problems facing older adults, including abuse, are increasing each year. Elder abuse is generally defined as harmful acts toward an older adult, such as physical, sexual, and emotional or psychological abuse, as well as financial exploitation and neglect, including self-neglect. An average of 2,150,000 cases of elder abuse are reported each year (The National Center on Elder Abuse, Bureau of Justice Statistics, 2014). It is also suspected that there are an equal number of cases not reported each year, and that an estimated 9.5% of older adults will experience some type of abuse. In 2014, the National Center on Elder Abuse found that 91% of nursing homes lack adequate staff to properly care for residents and that 36% of nursing homes violate elder abuse laws each year. Consequences of elder abuse are generally criminal in nature. Sometimes a facility will be fined or, in extreme cases, lose its license for repeated acts of abuse.

Bullying is not included in the definition of elder abuse, and there are no federal laws that directly address the issue of bullying among older adults (U.S. Department of Health and Human Services, 2014). Although little to no research exists on bullying among older adults, Robin Bonifas estimates that 10%–20% of residents in older adult environments may be the targets of bullying (R. Bonifas, personal communication, 2015). Fortunately, society has begun to recognize that this population is not as able to protect and advocate for themselves. With this recognition comes the responsibility to put systematic protections in place and educate professionals in an effort to protect some of our most vulnerable citizens from being the targets of bullying.

In doing research for the Senior Culture program discussed in Chapter 8, I found that the biggest obstacle to awareness of the problem of bullying is a lack of self-reporting. Older adults seem not to report incidents of having witnessed someone being bullied due to a fear of retaliation, disbelief, and an overall feeling of not wanting to "create a problem." I asked many residents who shared their experiences of being bullied why they did not report the incident, and the response most often given was "I want to live the rest of my life out in peace, I am afraid of what will happen to me if I report it." As mentioned in previous chapters, we already know that the effects of bullying can be devastating and that the targets often experience loneliness, self-isolation, depression, and anxiety and may shut down or retreat emotionally. Securing a trusting relationship with residents is an essential first step in encouraging the reporting of bullying incidents. During the piloting of the Senior Culture program, participants felt more at ease in sharing information as conversations continued over several lessons and they became comfortable with the presenter. In addition, it is just as important to gain a clear understanding of what older adults know about bullying among people their age. When I first began piloting the Senior Culture program and defined and described bullying as it relates to older people, I watched the surprised looks from participants and listened to them make comments such as "Do old people really bully?" and "We don't have any of that happening here!" As the group began to understand better what bullying looks and feels like, a very different climate filled the room. Participants began to describe their personal experiences of bullying openly and, more important, they seemed to experience a sense of empowerment and freedom.

In piloting the Senior Culture program, I found that underreporting of bullying incidents also seems to be a contributing factor to a lack of awareness of the issue on the part of caregiving staff, healthcare professionals, and organization administration. Conversely, administrators have expressed concerns about how their reputation and bottom line will be affected by acknowledging and implementing ways to prevent bullying behaviors among residents. What regulations and laws may be obstacles to protecting the targets, such as evicting the bully or firing employees? Will instituting interventions result in a negative reputation for the facility and will it lose residents? These concerns can be overcome by increasing awareness among all staff and professionals who work with older adults to tackle the epidemic of bullying from all directions.

A Systematic Response of Intervention and Prevention

Increased awareness will also lead to a greater push for prevention programming as well as legislation. Appropriate legislation could be modeled on laws created to protect children against bullying. Although the laws vary for children by state, according to www.stopbullying.gov (2014) there are several key components to assist states in creating or improving anti-bullying laws.

Anti-bullying laws for children have a clear purpose, including recognition of the effects of bullying on students and their learning and safety. Laws to combat bullying among older adults should also have a clear purpose, including recognition of how it affects older adults' ability to feel safe and function effectively within their surroundings as well as the overall emotional climate of their community. The purpose statement should recognize that everyone who lives or works in a senior care setting must be engaged and responsible for preventing and remedying bullying and that administration, staff, and others working in or visiting the premises should be partners in a community effort to address bullying.

Anti-bullying laws designed for children contain a statement of the scope of the law; that is, where and when the law will apply and who will be subject to the law. For older adults, the scope of the law may not be easy to define. Thus, a clear and concise statement of the scope of the law will be critical. There also needs to be a clear statement regarding who will be subject to anti-bullying laws. Will the law apply to residents only, or will it be extended to visitors and family members? Will the law apply to all administrators and professionals working with the residents or just those employed by the facility? Finally, it will be important to determine what type of facilities will be subject to these laws. Will it apply to any facility that serves adults age 55 and older or just residential communities? Will it apply to both public and private programs? Will it apply to just those programs that receive state or federal funding or any service or program that requires a license by the county or state? Unlike with children, older adults maintain all of their independent rights. Most states have very strong laws against interfering with someone's rights just because they are getting older. Laws will need to strike a delicate balance between interfering with an independent adult's right to behave how they choose and protecting those who are most vulnerable to being bullied.

Anti-bullying laws for children have a clear definition of what types of behaviors are considered bullying. For example, most school districts require the behavior to be repetitive before it is labeled as bullying. However, because bullying among older adults can be more subtle, any definition within the statute must clearly define bullying behavior and indicate examples of specific behaviors to ensure that the behaviors are recognizable by all.

Anti-bullying laws for children define who may be at risk for being bullied. Specifically, certain characteristics such as race, gender, national origin, physical appearance, and sexual orientation have typically targeted children for being bullied. The laws also explain that bullying can happen to anyone and is not always based on any specific characteristic. Although laws related to older adults should contain this component, it is important to recognize that all older adults are at risk. The most at risk to specifically cite include those who are physically frail or emotionally vulnerable, those who use an assistive device such as a walker or a cane, those who have a memory problem, the poor, or those who do not have a supportive family.

Anti-bullying laws for children require the local educational agency (LEA) to develop and implement policies that prohibit bullying and take into account all parties of interest, including, but not limited to students, school administrators, teachers, and members of the community. Policies generally include definitions of bullying, the process for reporting an incident, investigation procedures, how written records are to be maintained, consequences and sanctions for bullying, and the process for referrals to mental health and other health professionals for both the target and the bully. Because there is no comparable agency for older adults, this is an important issue to address. What agency could serve as the local regulating agency for older adults? Each state appears to have some sort of senior services department or agency as well as some sort of regulatory agency for assisted living communities, skilled nursing facilities, and memory care units. Independent living facilities, however, are typically regulated by the hotel and restaurant management agencies and do not fall under the same stringent guidelines. In addition, retirement or 55+ communities, senior centers, places of worship, and any other location where older adults gather are not under the authority of these state senior regulating agencies. Any one of these agencies within each state would be a logical choice for coordinating efforts to define and implement policies that prohibit bullying.

Another important issue is ensuring that local agencies are implementing polices with fidelity. How will these local agencies be monitored? Who will assess their efficacy in reaching the legislation's goals? What data will be collected, and how will it be collected? For children, each state has a Department of Education that oversees the local educational agencies. Furthermore, the U.S. Department of Education oversees many aspects of states' department of education. There is currently no comparable hierarchy for older adults.

Another key component of anti-bullying laws for children is a clear plan to communicate the law's purpose and scope as well as the consequences for violating the law. The same procedure should be in place for older adults; that is, creating a uniform understanding of acceptable and unacceptable behaviors and a clear understanding of who will be subjected to these laws. A communication plan must include the dissemination of the information in several forms to residents, staff, and families, including posting in common areas, providing in both verbal and written format, posting on the company's website, and disseminating via in-services for staff and programming for residents and community members.

One of the most important components of anti-bullying laws for children is training and education. For older adults, this should also be of utmost importance. Training and education equip professionals to help identify, prevent, and manage bullying behaviors. This component should also address the implementation of resident- and community-based prevention programs.

Finally, child anti-bullying laws clearly state that targets may seek any type of legal action they wish and are not bound by any law preventing them from doing so. This means that any available civil or criminal claims can be brought against a perpetrator regardless of the consequences imposed by the anti-bullying laws. For example, the harshest penalty children face for bullying is expulsion from school. The legal action available to older adult targets will depend on the scope and nature of the consequences imposed by anti-bullying laws for older adults.

Recent Legislation

Legislators in Massachusetts proposed two bills in 2015 to address bullying among older adults in subsidized, multi-family housing developments. The first bill would provide for an in-depth study of the problem and identification of potential remedies. The second bill would require landlords and managers to help prevent and remedy bullying in the residential environment and was modeled after school anti-bullying laws. It not only identifies prohibited actions and penalties for infractions, but also creates a framework for training and education to encourage conformity among efforts to reduce and eliminate bullying. The second bill would also require landlords and managers to work with residents to develop plans, train and educate staff and residents, receive and act on reports of bullying, and discipline transgressors for infractions. Oversight would be provided by the Public Safety Division of the Commonwealth's Attorney General's Office. This office, in consultation with a number of agencies, experts, and citizens, would publish model plans to guide programs. Although these bills only address bullying in subsidized housing developments, they provide guidance on how to begin to address this problem in the broader community. Any proposed legislation must include staff administration trainings on the importance of building caring communities, creating a congruent climate, identifying and addressing inappropriate behaviors, and addressing bullying behaviors. There must also be ongoing programming for residents on issues such as prevention, managing bullying issues as they arise, and creating committees that include stakeholders.

Summary

Although research to date on bullying among older adults has revealed more questions than answers, it is clear that older adults are just as vulnerable as children to its negative effects and need the same legislative protections. A systematic response of intervention and prevention is needed to address this unseen epidemic, beginning with more education, research, and policies and procedures. Furthermore, existing legislation that addresses bullying among children can serve as a starting point for creating legislation to protect older adults.

Appendix

Social Interaction Survey

Your answers are confidential. Please try to answer the questions as honestly as you can.

1. What is your gender?

	Male
	Female

2. What is your age?

	59 years or younger
	60–69 years
	70–79 years
	80–89 years
	90–99 years
	100 years or older

3. What is your ethnicity?

	Latino/Hispanic
	Middle Eastern
	African
	Caribbean
	South Asian
	East Asian
	Caucasian
	Multiracial
	Other (please note)

(Adapted from the work of Rodney Pruitt, M.A. Used with permission.)

(Continued)

4. Do you feel safe in this community?

	Never
	Sometimes
	Often
	Always
	Additional comments

5. Do you feel safe in your room or apartment?

	Never
	Sometimes
	Often
	Always
	Additional comments

6. Do you feel safe on the way to and from activities?

	Never
	Sometimes
	Often
	Always
	Additional comments

(Continued)

~~~~~~

7. Do you feel safe in the dining room?

	Never
	Sometimes
	Often
	Always
	Additional comments

8. Have other residents interacted with you in the past 3 months in any of the following ways? (Check one answer for each question.)

Physically? (Examples: hit, pushed, slapped, kicked, had property stolen)

	Never
	One or two times
	Three or four times
	Every week
	Every day
	Additional comments

Verbally? (Examples: called names, teased, insulted, threatened)

	Never
	One or two times
	Three or four times
	Every week
	Every day
	Additional comments

(Continued)

~~~~~~

Socially? (Examples: excluded from a group, gossiped about, rumors spread about you)

	Never
	One or two times
	Three or four times
	Every week
	Every day
	Additional comments

Related to gender? (Examples: excluded or treated badly because you are a man or a woman; overheard sexist comments)

	Never
	One or two times
	Three or four times
	Every week
	Every day
	Additional comments

Related to disability? (Examples: excluded because of a difference in ability or because of an adaptive device, such as a walker or hearing aid)

	Never
	One or two times
	Three or four times
	Every week
	Every day
	Additional comments

(Continued)

9. **How often have you seen another resident being treated in any of the following ways in the past 3 months? (Check one answer for each question.)**

Physically? (Examples: hit, pushed, slapped, kicked, had property stolen)

	Never
	One or two times
	Three or four times
	Every week
	Every day
	Additional comments

Verbally? (Examples: called names, teased, insulted, threatened)

	Never
	One or two times
	Three or four times
	Every week
	Every day
	Additional comments

Socially? (Examples: excluded from a group, gossiped about, rumors spread about that person)

	Never
	One or two times
	Three or four times
	Every week
	Every day
	Additional comments

(Continued)

Related to gender? (Examples: excluded or treated badly because the resident is a man or a woman; overheard sexist comments)

	Never
	One or two times
	Three or four times
	Every week
	Every day
	Additional comments

Related to disability? (Examples: excluded because of a difference in ability or because of an adaptive device, such as a walker or hearing aid)

	Never
	One or two times
	Three or four times
	Every week
	Every day
	Additional comments

10. How often have you stayed away from common areas, such as the dining room, in order to avoid negative social interactions in the past 3 months?

	Never
	One or two times
	Three or four times
	Every week
	Every day
	Additional comments

(Continued)

11. **How often have you tried to help another resident who was involved in a negative social interaction?**

	Never
	One or two times
	Three or four times
	Every week
	Every day
	Additional comments

Where and how often do negative social interactions occur?	Never	Sometimes	Often	Always
At night (11 p.m. to 7 a.m.)				
During the day (7 a.m. to 3 p.m.)				
In the evening (3 p.m. to 11 p.m.)				
On the weekends				
In your room or apartment				
In the hallways				
During activities				
In the dining room				
In the rehabilitation room				
In the laundry room				
In the parking lot				
Other (please note)				

(Continued)

~~~~~~

Think of the last time you saw another resident experience a negative social interaction. What did you do? (Check all that apply.)

	I have not seen another resident experience a negative social interaction.
	I ignored it.
	I told my family about it.
	I told my aide about it.
	I told the nurse about it.
	I told the social worker about it.
	I told an administrator or supervisor about it.
	I told another staff member about it.
	I told another resident about it.
	At the time, I helped the person.
	Later on, I helped the person.
	I watched.
	I made a joke about it.
	I joined in on the interaction.
	I got someone to help stop it.
	I stood up to the person who was doing it.
	I got back at the person who was doing it later.
	Other (please explain):

(Continued)

People are often reluctant to intervene when they see another person being treated negatively in a social interaction. If you chose not to intervene when you saw someone experience a negative social interaction, what prompted that choice? (Check the 3 answers that apply the most.)

	I didn't want to get involved.
	I was afraid.
	I didn't know what to do or who to talk to.
	I thought if I told someone, they wouldn't do anything about it.
	It isn't right to tell on other people.
	The social interaction wasn't so bad.
	The person who was experiencing it deserved it.
	I do not like the person who experienced it.
	It wasn't my business or my problem.
	I didn't want to get in trouble for telling.
	I did not want to become a target also.
	Other (please explain):

What can staff members and the administration do to help stop negative social interactions? (Check the 3 answers that apply the most.)

	Enforce the rules we use.
	Make new rules.
	Supervise better.
	Teach social skills.
	Teach residents about negative social interactions and ways to stop it.
	Teach staff members about negative social interactions and ways to stop it.

(Continued)

	Create a form so residents can make a report anonymously.
	Make the consequences for negative social interactions more severe.
	Other (please explain):

Is there anything else about negative social interactions you would like to share with us?

Is there anything we could do to make our community a safer or nicer place to be?

Bullying Incident Report Form

〰〰〰〰〰〰〰〰〰〰〰〰〰〰〰〰〰〰〰〰〰〰〰〰〰〰〰

Name of reporter/person filing the report:

_____

(Leave blank if report is being filed anonymously)

Check whether you are the: ❏ Target of the behavior   ❏ Reporter

Check whether you are a:

❏ Resident   ❏ Staff member (specify role) _____

❏ Visitor   ❏ Other (specify) _____

Contact information _____

Date of incident _____ Time of incident _____

Location of incident _____

Information about the incident:

Name(s) of target(s) of behavior: _____

Name(s) of person(s) who engaged in the behavior: _____

Name(s) of witnesses: _____

Please describe what happened, including names of people involved, what occurred, and what
each person said and did. Use additional space on the back, if needed.

_____

_____

_____

_____

(Adapted from the work of Rodney Pruitt, M.A. Used with permission.)

(Continued)

Bullying Incident Report Form *continued*

Bullying incident related to (check all that apply):

❏ Age   ❏ Disabilities   ❏ Health condition   ❏ Sexual orientation

❏ Race   ❏ Gender   ❏ Appearance   ❏ Religion or culture

❏ Other (please describe) _____

Form of bullying (check all that apply):

❏ Physical aggression   ❏ Deliberately excluding   ❏ Verbal threats

❏ Name calling and taunting   ❏ Damaging or taking personal possessions

❏ Spreading rumors   ❏ Extortion

❏ Other (please describe): _____

_____

_____

_____

_____

Signature of person filing form (if not filing anonymously):

_____ Date: _____

References

Alcon, A., Burnes, K., & Frankel, M. (March, 2014). *Social bullying: Training older adults to make a positive difference.* Workshop presentation at the American Society on Aging, Aging in American Conference, San Diego, California.

Algase, D. L, Beck, C., Kolawnowski, A., Whall, A., Berent, S., Richards, K., & et al. (1996). Need-driven dementia-compromised behavior (NDB): An alternative view of disruptive behavior. *American Journal of Alzheimer's Disease and Other Dementias, 5*, 10–19.

American Senior Housing Association. (2014). *Unlocking the mystery behind very satisfied independent living customers: Make them "feel at home."* Washington, DC: American Senior Housing Association.

Altman, B. A. (2010). Workplace bullying: Application of Novak's (1998) learning theory and implications for training. *Employee Responsibilities and Rights Journal, 22*(1), 21–32.

Anderson, S. A. (March 3, 2011). Mickey Rooney: I was abused. Available at http://www.huffingtonpost.com/2011/03/03/mickey-rooney-i-was-abuse_n_830897.html

Axelrod, J. (June 22, 2012). Karen Klein's school bus bullies receive death threats. Available at http://www.cbsnews.com/8301-505263_162-57458574/karen-kleins-school-bus-bullies-receive-death-threats/

Batsche, G. M., & Knoff, H. M. (1994). Bullies and their victims. Understanding a pervasive problem in the schools. *School Psychology Review, 23*, 165–175.

Beddoe, A. E., & Murphy, S. O. (2004). Does mindfulness decrease stress and foster empathy among nursing students? *Journal of Nursing Education, 43*(7), 305–312.

Bonifas, R. P. (January, 2014). Relational aggression in assisted living facilities: Insights into an under-recognized phenomenon. Paper presentation at the 18th Annual Conference of the Society for Social Work Research, San Antonio, Texas.

Bjorkqvist, K., Ekman, K., & Lagerspetz, K. (1982). Bullies and victims: Their ego picture, ideal ego picture and normative ego picture. *Scandinavian Journal of Psychology, 23*, 307–313.

Bonifas, R. P. (2011). Understanding challenging social relationships in senior housing communities. Unpublished raw data; Arizona State University, Phoenix, Arizona.

Bonifas, R. P., & Kramer, C. (November, 2011). Senior bullying in assisted living: Residents' perspectives. Poster presentation at the 64th Annual Scientific Meeting of the Gerontological Society of America, Boston, Massachusetts.

Bonifas, R. P., & Frankel, M. (March, 2012). Is it bullying? Strategies for assessing and intervening with older adults. Workshop presentation at the Aging in America Conference of the American Society on Aging, Washington, D.C.

Bonifas, R. P., & Hector, P. (2013). Senior bullying in assisted living: Insights into an underrecognized phenomenon. *Journal of the American Medical Directors' Association, 14*(3), B25–26.

Bradshaw, C. P., Sawyer, A. L., & O'Brennan, L. M. (2007). Bullying and peer victimization at school: Perceptual differences between students and school staff. *School Psychology Review, 36*(3), 361–382.

Forni, P. M. (2002). *Choosing civility: Twenty-five tools of considerate conduct.* New York: Saint Martin's Press.

Creno, C. (December 28, 2010). Chandler woman, 76, experiences bullying. *Arizona Republic.*

Cunico, L., Sartori, R., Marognolli, O., & Meneghini, A. M. (2012). Developing empathy in nursing students: A cohort longitudinal study. *Journal of Clinical Nursing, 21,* 2016–2025.

Decety, J., & Moriguchi, Y. (2007). The empathic brain and its dysfunction in psychiatric populations: Implications for intervention across different clinical conditions. *BioPyschoSocial Medicine, 1,* 1–21.

Duluth Superior Area Community Foundation. (n.d.). Common Resolution Document. Available at http://www.dsaspeakyourpeace.org.

Fredriksen-Goldsen, K. I., Kim, H. J., Emlet, C. A., Muraco, A., Erosheva, E. A., Hoy-Ellis, C.P., . . . Petry, H. (2011). *The aging and health report: Disparities and resilience among lesbian, gay, bisexual, and transgender older adults.* Seattle, WA: Institute for Multigenerational Health.

Gerdes, K. E., & Segal, E. A. (2009). A social work model of empathy. *Advances in Social Work, 10,* 114–127.

Gray, M. J., Litz, B. T., Hsu, J. L., & Lombardo, T. W. (2004). Psychometric properties of the Life Events Checklist. *Assessment, 11*(4), 330–341.

Hawker, S. S. J., & Boulton, M. J. (2000). Twenty years' research on peer victimization and psychosocial maladjustment: A meta-analytic review of cross-sectional studies. *Journal of Child Psychology and Psychiatry, 41,* 441–455.

Hawkins, D. L., Pepler, D., & Craig, W. M. (2001). Peer interventions in playground bullying. *Social Development, 10,* 512–527.

Hazelden Foundation. (2011). Bullying is a serious issue. Available at http://www.violencepreventionworks.org/public/bullying.page

Hirano, M., & Yukawa, S. (2014). Relationship between mindfulness and anger: Focusing on multidimensionality of mindfulness tendency. *Personality and Individual Differences, 60.* doi:10.1016/j.paid.2013.07.111

Ireland, J., & Archer, J. (2004). Association between measures of aggression and bullying among juvenile and young offenders. *Aggressive Behavior, 30,* 29–42.

Jolliffe, D., & Farrington, D. P. (2004). Empathy and offending: A systematic review and meta-analysis. *Aggression and Violent Behavior, 9,* 441–476.

Kabat-Zinn, J. (1994). *Wherever you go, there you are: Mindfulness meditation in everyday life.* New York: Hyperion.

Kessler, J. (December 11, 2009). Woman, 98, indicted in death of 100-year-old nursing home roommate. Available at http://articles.cnn.com/2009-12-11/justice/nursing.home.killing_1_nursing-home-roommate-competency-evaluation-elizabeth-barrow?_s=PM:CRIME

Kosciw, J. G., Greytak, E. A., Bartkiewicz, M. J., Boesen, M. J., & Palmer, N. A. (2012). The 2011 National School Climate Survey: The experiences of lesbian, gay, bisexual and transgender youth in our nation's schools. New York: GLSEN.

Lachs, M., Bachman, R., Williams, C. S., & O'Leary, J. R. (2007). Resident-to-resident elder mistreatment and police contact in nursing homes: Findings from a population-based cohort. *Journal of the American Geriatrics Association, 55*, 840–845.

Leff, S. S., & Waasdorp, T. E. (2013). Effect of aggression and bullying on children and adolescents: Implications for prevention and intervention. *Current Psychiatry Reports, 15*(3), 343.

Lessne, D., & Harmalkar, S. (2013). Student reports of bullying and cyber-bullying: Results from the 2011 School Crime Supplement to the National Crime Victimization Survey. Available at https://nces.ed.gov/pubs2013/2013329.pdf.

Liefooghe, A. P. D., & Mackenzie Davey, K. (2003). Explaining bullying at work: Why should we listen to employee accounts? In S. Einarsen, H. Hoel, D. Zapf & C. L. Cooper (Eds.), *Bullying and emotional abuse in the workplace: International perspectives in research and practice* (pp. 219–230). London: Taylor & Francis.

Mapes, D. (February 16, 2011). Mean old girls: Seniors who bully. Available at http://www.nbcnews.com/id/41353544/ns/health-aging/t/mean-old-girls-seniors-who-bully/#.V07tdGZ9grc

McBee, L. (2008). *Mindfulness-based elder care: A CAM model for frail elders and their caregivers.* New York: Springer Publisher Company.

Moon, B., McCluskey, J., & Schreck, C. (2013). School bullying and victimization. *Journal of Criminology.* doi:10.1155/2013/626317

Napoli, M., Krech, P., & Holley, L. (2005). Mindfulness practice training for elementary school students: The Attention Academy Program. *Journal of Applied School Psychology, 21*, 99–125.

Nasreddine Z. S., Phillips, N. A., Bédirian, V., Charbonneau, S., Whitehead, V., Collin, I., Cummings, J. L., & et al. (2005). The Montreal cognitive assessment, MoCA: A brief screening tool for mild cognitive impairment. *Journal of the American Geriatrics Society, 53*, 695–699.

National Center on Elder Abuse. (2006). The 2004 survey of state adult protective services: Abuse of adults 60 years of age an older. Available at http://www.elderabusecenter.org/pdf/2-14-06%20FINAL%2060+REPORT.pdf

National Center on Elder Abuse. (2011). What is elder abuse? Available at http://www.ncea.aoa.gov/Main_Site/FAQ/Questions.aspx

Nay, R. (1995). Nursing home residents' perceptions of relocation. *Journal of Clinical Nursing, 4*, 319–325.

Newman, K., & Roberts, J. (2001). Bring a dish to pass: The civil action of community. Muscatine, IA: National Civility Center.

Novak, J. D. (1998). *Learning, creating, and using knowledge: Concept maps™ as facilitative tools in schools and corporations.* Mahwah, NJ: Lawrence Erlbaum.

Olweus, D. (1991). Bully/victim problems among school children: Basic facts and effects of a school based intervention program. In I. Rubin & D. Pepler (Eds.), *The development and treatment of childhood aggression,* pp. 411–447. Hillsdale, NJ: Erlbaum.

Olweus, D. (1993). *Bullying at school: What we know and what we can do.* Oxford: Blackwell.

Pardasani, M. (2010). Senior centers: Characteristics of participants and nonparticipants. *Activities, Adaptation, & Aging, 34*, 48–70.

Pengpid, S., & Peltzer, K. (2013). Bullying and its associated factors among school-aged adolescents in Thailand. *The Scientific World Journal,* doi:10.1155/2013/254083

Purcell, M., & Murphy, J. (2014). *Mindfulness for teen anger: A workbook to overcome anger and aggression using MBSR and DBT skills.* Oakland, CA: New Harbinger Publications.

Rayner, C., & Keashly, L. (2005). Bullying at work: A perspective from Britain and North America. In S. Fox & P. E. Spector (Eds.), *Counterproductive work behavior: Investigations of actors and targets* (pp. 271–296). Washington, DC: American Psychological Association.

Reese, R. (March 22, 2012). Georgia woman, 87, accused of bullying neighbor. Available at http://abcnews.go.com/blogs/headlines/2012/03/georgia-woman-87-accused-of-bullying-neighbor/

Rex-Lear, M. (2011). *Not just a playground issue: Bullying among older adults and the effects on their individual health.* Unpublished doctoral dissertation, University of Texas at Arlington.

Rice, G. E. (February 3, 2014). Bullying knows no age limit, warn experts who see a rise in cases among seniors. *The Kansas City Star.* Available at http://www.kansascity.com/news/local/article338209/Bullying-knows-no-age-limit-warn-experts-who-see-a-rise-in-cases-among-seniors.html

Riess, K., Kelley, J. M., Bailey, R. W., Dunn, E. J., & Phillips, M. (2012). Empathy training for resident physicians: A randomized controlled trial of a neuroscience-informed curriculum. *Journal of General Internal Medicine, 27,* 1280–1286.

Richardson, D., Hommock, G., Smith, S., Gardner, W., & Manuel, S. (1994). Empathy as a cognitive inhibitor of interpersonal aggression. *Aggressive Behavior, 20,* 275–289.

Rosenberg, M. (2003). *Nonviolent communication.* Encinitis, CA: PuddleDancer Press.

Sahin, M. (2012). An investigation into the efficiency of empathy training program on preventing bullying in primary schools. *Children and Youth Services Review, 34,* 1325–1330.

Saunders, P., Huynh, A., & Goodman-Delahunty, J. (2007). Defining workplace bullying behavior professional lay definitions of workplace bullying. *International Journal of Law and Psychiatry, 30,* 340–354.

Saleebey, D. (2006). *The strengths perspective in social work practice.* New York: Allyn & Bacon.

Shinoda–Tagawa, T., Leonard, R., Pontikas, J., McDonough, J., Allen, D., & Dreyer, P. (2004). Resident-to-resident violent incidents in nursing homes. *Journal of the American Medical Association, 291,* 591–598.

Siegel, D. J. (2007) *The mindful brain: Reflection and attunement in the cultivation of well-being.* New York: W.W. Norton and Co.

Smith, R. (December 14, 2009). 98-year-old Laura Lindquist murdered 100-year-old nursing home roommate Elizabeth Barrow, say cops. Available at http://www.cbsnews.com/8301-504083_162-5968100-504083.html

Smith, P. K., & Brain, P. (2000). Bullying in schools: Lessons from two decades of research. *Aggressive Behaviour, 26,* 1–9.

Trompetter, H., Scholte, R., & Westerhof, G. (2011). Resident-to-resident relational aggression and subjective well-being in assisted living facilities. *Aging and Mental Health, 15,* 59–67.

Ttofi, M. M., & Farrington, D. P. (2011). Effectiveness of school-based programs to reduce bullying: A systematic and meta-analytic review. *Journal of Experimental Criminology, 7*(1), 27–56.

Walker, S., & Richardson, D. R. (1998). Aggression strategies among older adults: Delivered but not seen. *Aggression and Violent Behavior, 3,* 287–294.

Wang, J., Iannotti, R. J., & Nansel, T. R. (2009). School bullying among adolescents in the United States: Physical, verbal, relational, and cyber. *Journal of Adolescent Health, 45*(4), 368–375.

Wood, F. (2007). *Bullying in nursing homes: Prevalence and consequences to psychological health.* Minneapolis, MN: Walden University.

Zapf, D., Einarsen, S., Hoel, H., & Vartia, M. (2003). Empirical findings on bullying in the workplace. In S. Einarsen, H. Hoel, D. Zapf, & C. Cooper (Eds.), *Bullying and emotional abuse in the workplace. International perspectives in research and practice* (pp. 103–126). London: Taylor & Francis.

Resources

Anti-Defamation League
www.adl.org

Al-Anon Family Groups
www.al-anon.org

Alcoholics Anonymous
www.aa.org

Alzheimer's Association
www.alz.org

American Association of Retired Persons
www.aarp.org

Bully Lab
www.bullylab.com

Bully Prevention Alliance
www.bpindyinc.org

CDC Violence Prevention
www.cdc.gov/violenceprevention

Character Matters
www.charactermattersnc.com

Creating Cultures of Dignity
www.rosalindwiseman.com

Cyber Bullying Resource Center
www.cyberbullying.us

Different Like Me
www.differentlikeme.com

My Better Nursing Home
www.mybetternursinghome.com

National Alliance on Mental Illness
www.nami.org

National Bullying Prevention Program
www.pacer.org

National Education Association
www.nea.org/bullyfree

Olweus Bullying Prevention Program
www.violencepreventionworks.org

Peers Social Skills Training Intervention
www.semel.ucla.edu/peers

Prevent Bullying in Society
www.bullying.org

Safe School Ambassadors Program
www.community-matters.org

Words Can Change Your Brain Neuroscience
www.markrobertwaldman.com

Work Place Bullying and Trauma Institute
www.workplacebullying.org

Index

~~~~~~

Note *b* indicates boxes, *f* figures, and *t* tables.